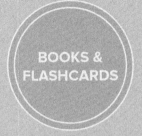
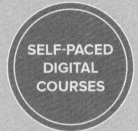
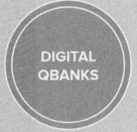
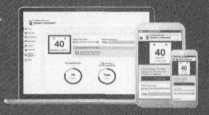

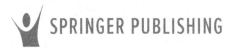

C-EFM®
CERTIFICATION
EXPRESS REVIEW

C-EFM®
CERTIFICATION
EXPRESS REVIEW

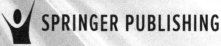

SPRINGER PUBLISHING

Springer Publishing Company, LLC
11 West 42nd Street, New York, NY 10036
www.springerpub.com

Acquisitions Editor: Elizabeth Nieginski
Compositor: diacriTech

ISBN: 978-0-8261-5877-2
ebook ISBN: 978-0-8261-5878-9
DOI: 10.1891/9780826158789

Printed by BnT

Library of Congress Control Number: 2022904195

Contact sales@springerpub.com to receive discount rates on bulk purchases.

Printed in the United States of America.

CONTENTS

Preface   ix
Pass Guarantee   xi

1   GENERAL EXAMINATION INFORMATION   *1*

Overview   *1*
Certification Requirements   *1*
About the Examination   *1*
How to Apply   *2*
How to Recertify   *2*
How to Contact National Certification Corporation   *3*

2   MATERNAL–FETAL OXYGENATION: PHYSIOLOGY AND PATHOPHYSIOLOGY   *5*

Maternal–Fetal Oxygenation   *5*
Resources   *7*

3   MONITORING EQUIPMENT AND ASSESSMENT METHODS   *9*

Electronic Fetal Monitoring   *9*
Electronic Fetal Monitoring Equipment   *10*
Uterine Activity Assessment   *13*
Fetal Assessment Methods   *15*
Resources   *23*

4   ELECTRONIC FETAL MONITORING PATTERN RECOGNITION   *25*

Categories of Fetal Heart Rate Tracings   *25*
Fetal Heart Rate Baseline   *27*
Fetal Heart Rate Variability   *28*
Fetal Heart Rate Accelerations   *32*
Fetal Heart Rate Decelerations   *34*
Fetal Arrythmias   *42*
Resources   *46*

5   COMPLICATIONS   *47*

Fetal Complications   *47*

Environmental Conditions   *47*

Maternal Respiratory System   *48*

Maternal Lungs   *48*

Maternal Blood Flow   *48*

Maternal Cardiac Disease and Blood Disorders   *48*
Maternal Hypotension   *49*
Hypertensive Disorders in Pregnancy   *50*
Maternal Hypovolemia and Hemorrhage   *53*
Inferior Vena Cava Compression   *55*

Maternal Seizure   *56*

Uterus   *58*

Uterine Rupture   *58*
Excessive Uterine Activity (Tachysystole)   *59*

Placenta   *60*

Abruptio Placenta   *60*
Placental Implantation Complications   *61*

Umbilical Cord   *62*

Nuchal Cord   *62*
Umbilical Cord Compression   *63*
Umbilical Cord Prolapse   *64*

Fetus   *65*

Hypoxia/Acidosis   *65*
Shoulder Dystocia   *67*

Other Maternal Complications   *69*

Chorioamnionitis   *69*
Postpartum Hemorrhage   *70*
Diabetes Mellitus   *71*
Obesity   *72*

Complications of Labor   *73*

Failure to Progress   *73*
Operative Delivery   *73*
Preterm Labor   *74*
Resources   *75*

6   PROFESSIONAL ISSUES   *77*

Overview   *77*
Ethics   *77*
Legality   *79*
Patient Safety   *81*
Quality Improvement   *83*
Resources   *84*

7 TRACINGS ANALYSIS PRACTICE *87*

Patient Case Studies *87*
Resources *126*

8 POP QUIZ ANSWERS *127*

Appendix: Abbreviations *131*
Index *133*

PREFACE

If you have purchased this *Express Review*, you are likely well into your exam prep journey to certification. This book has been designed to be a high-speed review—a last-minute gut check before your exam day. We created this review, which is a quick summary of the key topics you'll encounter on the exam, to supplement your certification preparation studies. We encourage you to use it in conjunction with other study aids to ensure you are as prepared as possible for the exam.

This book follows the National Certification Corporation's (NCC) most recent exam content outline. It uses a succinct, bulleted format with sample EFM tracings to highlight essential knowledge. The aim of this book is to help you solidify your retention of information in the month or so leading up to your exam. It is written by certified nurse practitioners who are familiar with the exam and the content you need to know. Special features appear throughout the book to call out important information, including the following:

- Complications: Problems that can arise with certain patient conditions or procedures
- Nursing Pearls: Additional patient care insights and strategies for knowledge retention
- Alerts: Need-to-know details on how to handle emergency situations or when to transfer care
- Pop Quizzes: Critical thinking questions to test your ability to synthesize what you learned (answers in Chapter 8)
- List of Abbreviations: A useful appendix to help guide you through the alphabet soup of clinical terms

We know life is busy. Being able to prepare for your exam efficiently and effectively is paramount, which is why we created this *Express Review*. You have come to the right place as you continue on your path of professional growth and development. The stakes are high, and we want to help you succeed. Best of luck to you on your certification journey. You've got this!

PASS GUARANTEE

If you use this resource to prepare for your exam and you do not pass, you may return it for a refund of your full purchase price. To receive a refund, you must return your product along with a copy of your original receipt and exam score report. Product must be returned and received within 180 days of the original purchase date. Excludes tax, shipping, and handling. One offer per person and address. Refunds will be issued within 8 weeks from acceptance and approval. This offer is valid for U.S. residents only. Void where prohibited. To begin the process, please contact customer service at CS@springerpub.com.

1

GENERAL EXAMINATION INFORMATION

OVERVIEW

- The National Certification Corporation, founded in 1975 as a not-for-profit organization, offers multiple specialty certifications, including the subspecialty certification in EFM. EFM is a tool that provides the bedside clinician with real-time data concerning the status of both the pregnant patient and the fetus. Safety and quality of inpatient care are central to the mission of healthcare institutions, and EFM-certified healthcare professionals show commitment to their education and expertise and to providing optimal care.

CERTIFICATION REQUIREMENTS

- C-EFM® applicants must hold current, active, and unencumbered licensure in the United States or Canada as a physician, RN, nurse practitioner, nurse midwife or midwife, physician assistant, or paramedic.

ABOUT THE EXAMINATION

- This certification is offered via computer at a computer test center or at home with live remote proctoring.
- The National Certification Corporation provides a content outline for the C-EFM examination on its website that includes the percentage distribution of questions per each major content category. This is included as part of the National Certification Corporation Candidate Guide: Electronic Fetal Monitoring C-EFM®, which is updated annually.
- The 2-hour computer-based certification examination contains up to 125 test questions; 100 of the questions are scored and the other 25 questions are included as pretest items. The pretest items do not impact the final score of the assessment. All questions are multiple choice with a premise and three possible answers.
- The 125 questions are broken down into the following categories:
  - Electronic monitoring equipment (5%)
    - External and internal
    - Artifact
    - Signal ambiguity
    - Failure
    - Troubleshooting

(continued)

ABOUT THE EXAMINATION *(continued)*

- Physiology (11%)
  - Uteroplacental factors affecting fetal oxygenation
- Pattern recognition and intervention (70%)
  - Fetal heart rate baseline
  - Fetal heart rate variability
  - Abnormal uterine activity
  - Fetal dysrhythmias
  - Maternal complications
  - Uteroplacental complications
  - Fetal complications
  - Fetal heart rate accelerations
  - Fetal heart rate decelerations
  - Normal uterine activity
- Fetal assessment methods (9%)
  - Auscultation
  - Fetal movement and stimulation
  - Nonstress testing
  - Biophysical profile
  - Cord blood and acid–base balance
- Professional issues (5%)
  - Legal
  - Ethics
  - Patient safety
  - Quality improvement

HOW TO APPLY

- Applications for the exam are accepted online only on the National Certification Corporation website. The National Certification Corporation sends application confirmation via email, and it can take from 1 to 14 days to process, review, and approve applications.
- Once approved, applicants have 90 days from the date of the application to take the exam and must schedule the exam within the first 30 days of the eligibility window.
- The exam cost is $210, including a $50 application fee.

HOW TO RECERTIFY

The National Certification Corporation certification must be maintained every 3 years. Certification that is not maintained will expire. The National Certification Corporation certification maintenance program allows certification holders to continue certification status by obtaining 15 hours of continuing education credit. For continuing education credit to be used for certification maintenance, it must be earned between the date of notification of certification and the date maintenance is due.

HOW TO CONTACT NATIONAL CERTIFICATION CORPORATION

Website: nccwebsite.org
Email address: info@nccnet.org

Mailing address:
National Certification Corporation
676 N. Michigan Avenue, Suite 3600
Chicago, IL 60611

2

MATERNAL–FETAL OXYGENATION: PHYSIOLOGY AND PATHOPHYSIOLOGY

- Fetal oxygenation collectively depends on adequate maternal oxygenation; a healthy, functioning placenta; adequate maternal blood flow and volume; and adequate umbilical circulation.
- Three phases of oxygenation must occur to oxygenate the fetus:
  - There must be adequate oxygenation of the pregnant patient.
    - To stabilize maternal–fetal oxygen status, the nurse should change the position of the patient, administer an IV fluid bolus, and administer supplemental oxygen as needed.
  - The patient must pass oxygenated blood to the placenta. At the placenta, satisfactory gas exchange must occur.
  - The oxygenated blood is then transferred to the fetus via the umbilical cord.
- Fetal circulation:
  - As described earlier, oxygen-rich blood flows from maternal circulation to fetal circulation via the placenta to the umbilical cord.
  - The umbilical vein passes through the fetal liver and then splits.
  - Most of the oxygenated blood passes through a shunt, the ductus venosus, where it is taken to the inferior vena cava and then enters the right side of the fetal heart (Figure 2.1).
- Fetal heart:
  - Oxygen-rich blood flows through one of the two connections in the fetal heart: the foramen ovale and the ductus arteriosus.
    - The *foramen ovale* is an opening between the right and left atria that allows blood to bypass the lungs while the fetus is receiving oxygen from the placenta. This opening typically closes 6 months to 1 year after birth.
    - The *ductus arteriosus* is a blood vessel that connects the aorta and the pulmonary artery used to carry blood away from the lungs to the body. This vessel typically closes within a few days after birth.
  - The foramen ovale allows oxygen-rich blood to go from the right atrium to the left atrium, and then to the left ventricle and out the aorta to the brain. The blood circulates through the brain and arms, and then returns to the right atrium through the superior vena cava. Very little of this blood mixes with the oxygenated blood. This blood then enters the right ventricle.

(continued)

5

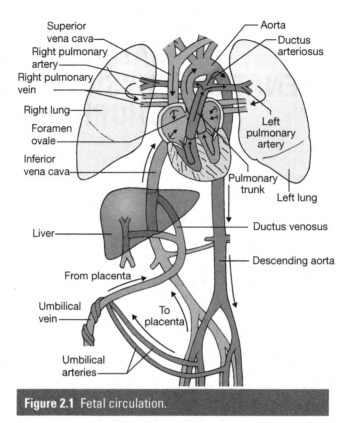

Figure 2.1 Fetal circulation.

Source: Jnah, A. J., & Trembath, A. N. (2018). *Fetal and neonatal physiology for the advanced practice nurse.* Springer Publishing Company.

MATERNAL–FETAL OXYGENATION
(continued)

- The less-oxygenated blood leaves the right ventricle through the aorta, where a small amount travels to the lungs. The rest of the blood is shunted through the ductus arteriosus to the descending aorta. This allows for oxygen-poor blood to leave the fetus through the umbilical cord arteries and return to the placenta to receive oxygen.
- Oxygen follows the steps in the maternal–fetal pathway to transfer from the environment, through the maternal body systems and essential organs, to the fetus. There can be interruptions at any step along the pathway, affecting fetal oxygenation (Table 2.1).

 ALERT!

Once the oxygenated blood is delivered to the fetus, the blood enters the fetal circulation.

 COMPLICATIONS

Interruptions of normal oxygen transfer can occur at any point along the maternal–fetal oxygenation pathway and cause fetal distress or demise.

 POP QUIZ 2.1

What interventions can be implemented by the nurse to improve uteroplacental circulation?

Table 2.1 Oxygen Pathway and Possible Interruptions

Steps for Oxygen Transfer from Environment to Fetus	Possible Interruptions Affecting Fetal Oxygenation at Each Point on the Pathway
1. Environmental conditions	Alteration in normal maternal respirations of 21% oxygenated air
2. Maternal respiratory system	Impaired gas exchange
3. Maternal blood flow	Decreased cardiac output
4. Maternal vasculature	Impaired blood flow
5. Uterus	Uterine contractions or injury
6. Placenta	Disruption of maternal/fetal gas exchange
7. Umbilical cord	Compression or injury
8. Fetus	Fetal response to interruptions in the oxygen pathway includes consequences such as hypoxia and fetal injury

RESOURCES

Ahmed, W. A. S., & Hamdy, M. A. (2018). Optimal management of umbilical cord prolapse. *International Journal of Women's Health, 10,* 459–465. https://doi.org/10.2147/IJWH.S130879

American College of Obstetricians and Gynecologists. (2020). Gestational hypertension and preeclampsia. *Obstetrics & Gynecology, 135*(6). https://doi.org/10.1097/aog.0000000000003891

AmericanPregnancy.org. (2021). *Umbilical cord prolapse and compression.* https://americanpregnancy .org/healthy-pregnancy/pregnancy-complications/umbilical-cord-prolapse/

Castillo-Castrejon, M., & Powell, T. L. (2017). Placental nutrient transport in gestational diabetic pregnancies. *Frontiers in Endocrinology, 8*(306), 1–9. https://doi.org/10.3389/fendo.2017.00306

Children's Hospital of Philadelphia. (2014). *Blood circulation in the fetus and newborn.* Author. https://www.chop.edu/conditions-diseases/blood-circulation-fetus-and-newborn.

Kawakita, T., Huang, C. C., & Landy, H. J. (2018). Risk factors for umbilical cord prolapse at the time of artificial rupture of membranes. *AJP Reports, 8*(2), e89–e94. https://doi.org/10.1055/s-0038-16 49486

Mayo Clinic. (2021). *Preeclampsia.* https://www.mayoclinic.org/diseases-conditions/preeclampsia/ symptoms-causes/syc-20355745

Miller, L. A., Miller, D. A., & Cypher, R. L. (2017). *Mosby's pocket guide to fetal monitoring: A multidisciplinary approach.* Elsevier.

Murray, M., Huelsmann, G., & Koperski, N. (2019). *Essentials of fetal and uterine monitoring* (sec. 5). Springer Publishing Company.

Nye, R. (2019). *Essentials of fetal heart rate monitoring* (chap. 7). Springer Publishing Company.

Prescribers' Digital Reference. (n.d). Invanz [Drug Information]. *PDR Search.* https://www.pdr.net/ drug-information/invanz?druglabelid=359

Sholapurkar, S. L. (2018). *Myths at the core of intrapartum cardiotocography interpretation–Risks of false Ideology, prospect theory and way forward. Obstetrics, Gynecology and Reproductive Medicine.* https://www.researchgate.net/publication/334448517_Myths_at_the_core_of_Intrapartum_Cardi otocography_Interpretation_Risks_of_false_Ideology_Prospect_theory_and_way_forward_ Clinical_Obstetrics_Gynecology_and_Reproductive_Medicine

3

MONITORING EQUIPMENT AND ASSESSMENT METHODS

ELECTRONIC FETAL MONITORING

Overview

- EFM is a tool that provides the bedside clinician with real-time data regarding the status of both the patient and the fetus.
- EFM uses internal monitors, external monitors, or a combination to measure and record the heart rate of the fetus as well as the pattern of the patient's uterine contractions.
- A printout of the monitored data is known as the *EFM tracing.*

Sample Tracing Strip

Figure 3.1 explains the components of a sample EFM strip.

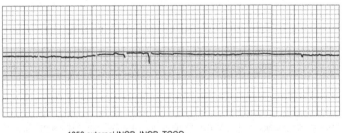

1950 external INOP INOP TOCO

Figure 3.1 Sample tracing strip. The intervals between the vertical lines represent 1 minute of monitoring. The fetal heart tracing is displayed in the upper pane, and uterine activity is displayed in the lower pane.

Source: Nye, R. (2019). *Essentials of fetal heart rate monitoring.* Springer Publishing Company.

ELECTRONIC FETAL MONITORING EQUIPMENT

Overview

- Fetal heart monitoring is a vital part of caring for a patient in labor. The RN must understand when, why, and how fetal monitoring equipment is used. Fetal monitoring equipment is important, but it is used *in addition to* the nurse's assessment, not as a replacement for a nurse assessment.
- Routine use of *continuous* fetal monitoring is not recommended for low-risk patients; however, *intermittent* fetal monitoring is appropriate for low-risk patients.
- Continuous fetal monitoring is considered appropriate for high-risk patients. Diagnoses considered at high risk include:
  - Maternal diabetes
  - Fetal defects
  - Maternal cardiac conditions
  - Preeclampsia
- There are two categories of EFM equipment:
  - External monitoring: ultrasound transducer
  - Internal monitoring: FSE
- There are two categories of potential issues with fetal monitoring equipment:
  - Artifact
  - Equipment failure

 ALERT!

A benefit of EFM is detection of early fetal distress resulting from fetal hypoxia and metabolic acidosis. Continuous fetal monitoring has been used to determine hypoxic-ischemic encephalopathy, cerebral palsy, and impending fetal death during labor. However, these events have a low prevalence, and continuous EFM has a false-positive rate of 99% in low-risk patients, which has been shown to increase the risk of cesarean section.

External Monitoring

- External monitoring typically requires patients to be physically connected to a monitor, which limits movement in labor. Some monitors offer wireless devices that can allow for movement, but these are not available in all facilities.
- Doppler ultrasound transducer
  - A monitor is placed on the patient's abdomen to continuously monitor FHR.
  - The ultrasound transducer sends sound waves and records the echoing waves of the FHR.
    - Measuring the echo waves determines how far away the object (i.e., the fetus) is, as well as the object's (i.e., the fetus's) size, shape, and consistency.
    - It is often used during prenatal visits and during labor to count the FHR.
- Fetoscope
  - A fetoscope is a type of stethoscope that is used to listen to, or auscultate, the FHR.
  - Place the fetoscope on the patient's abdomen to listen for the fetal heartbeat.
  - Count the FHR by using a timer or a watch or clock with a second hand. FHR is calculated in bpm.

- Tocodynamometer
  - A tocodynamometer is a pressure-sensitive device placed on the patient's abdomen over the uterus to measure uterine contractions.
  - It measures only when contractions occur and how long they last; their strength must be palpated.
  - It does not measure FHR, but it is required to determine the relationship between FHR and contractions.

Nursing Interventions

- Use Leopold's maneuver to locate the back of the fetus and place the ultrasound transducer on the patient's abdomen. For the best reading, the Doppler ultrasound transducer should be placed on the side of the patient's abdomen where the fetal back is located for the best reading.
- Move the transducer around the patient's abdomen until the FHR is heard the most loudly.
- If the FHR cannot be found, ask the patient where the FHR is normally found, or request bedside ultrasound by the OB provider to confirm location and presence of FHR.
- Use a band or strap to hold the ultrasound transducer in place.
- Place the tocodynamometer on the patient's fundus, where the contractions are most intense; it may need to be moved when the patient repositions.
- Document FHR assessment, any interventions, and patient response per facility policy.

 POP QUIZ 3.1

A patient requires an external monitoring device. The nurse cannot locate the FHR after moving the transducer around. The patient shows the nurse where the FHR is usually heard, but the nurse still cannot locate it. What should the nurse do next?

Internal Monitoring

- Internal monitors are inserted through a dilated cervix.
- Membranes must be ruptured in order to use an internal monitoring device.
- Patient movement is limited when connected to the monitor.
- Types of internal monitoring devices include:
  - FSE: An electrode inserted vaginally onto the fetal scalp that measures FHR. It must be inserted by a skilled provider.
  - IUPC: A catheter placed in the uterus to measure uterine contraction frequency, duration, strength, and resting tone. Using the IUPC is the only way to accurately measure strength of contractions using Montevideo units:

 NURSING PEARL

The strength of contractions is calculated by internally (not externally) measuring peak uterine pressure amplitude in mmHg, subtracting the resting tone of the contraction, and adding up the numbers in a 10-minute period. The peak resting tone × number of contractions in 10 minutes = x mmHg (Montevideo units).

 COMPLICATIONS

Because they require the amniotic sac to be broken, internal methods of fetal monitoring are invasive and can increase the risk of infection for the patient and fetus.

Internal Monitoring *(continued)*

- ○ Units are directly equal to pressure change in mmHg added up over a 10-minute period.
- ○ The IUPC measures only maternal uterine contractions, not FHR.
- ○ The IUPC may be needed to see contractions and their relationship to FHR.
- ○ The IUPC can be used to provide amnioinfusion.

Nursing Interventions

- Assist provider with equipment for FSE or IUPC.
- Assess and document, per institutional policy, the patient's heart rate, the FHR, any interventions, and the patient response.
- Follow and perform FHR assessments according to recommendations from professional organizations (including ACOG and AWHONN):
  - Low-risk patient: Every 15 to 30 minutes in labor, every 5 to 15 minutes while pushing
  - High-risk patient: Every 15 minutes in labor, every 5 minutes while pushing

Artifact

- Artifact occurs when there is a signal processing error. The fetal heart monitor recognizes and traces the patient's heart rate, not the FHR.
- Accelerations during pushing indicate that the fetal heart monitor is recognizing the patient's heart rate, not the FHR (Figure 3.2).
- FHR monitors have built-in autocorrelation algorithms that enable them to create a smooth FHR tracing.
- FHR may be absent due to fetal demise, so the FHR monitor may display the patient's heart rate instead.

Nursing Interventions

- Confirm fetal life before EFM with a bedside ultrasound.
- Measure the patient's pulse by continuous pulse oximetry while monitoring FHR.

 ALERT!

The nurse should advocate for an FSE when the fetus requires continuous monitoring and is difficult to monitor, as long as the cervix allows for insertion and membranes are ruptured.

 POP QUIZ 3.2

Given the benefits of EFM using internal methods, why does every pregnant patient not have an internal FSE to measure FHR?

 ALERT!

Accelerations that occur while pushing should alert the nurse that this may be the patient's heart rate rather than the FHR. Patient heart rate increases during the pushing stage of labor. The nurse should confirm FHR and patient heart rate to determine that there are two distinct heart rates. A pulse oximeter should be placed on the patient to determine patient heart rate; then an ultrasound should be used to determine FHR. It is important to rule out artifact to ensure that the FHR is accurately measured.

 ALERT!

Multiple-gestation FHRs may be similar, making it difficult to determine whether there are distinct FHRs. Nurses who cannot determine whether they are seeing the FHRs of separate fetuses should be prepared to call the provider for a bedside ultrasound to determine where each fetus's FHR is located.

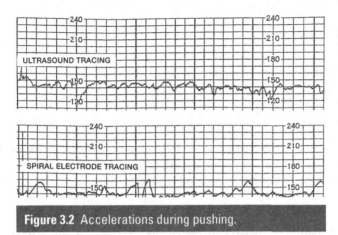

Figure 3.2 Accelerations during pushing.

Source: Murray, M., Huelsmann, G., & Koperski, N. (2019). *Essentials of fetal and uterine monitoring.* Springer Publishing Company.

Equipment Failure

- Fetal monitoring equipment can fail to work properly.
- Causes of failure include:
  - Equipment breaking
  - Power failure
  - Wrong equipment in use

Nursing Interventions

- Ensure proper equipment is used.
- Run a sample paper FHR tracing.
- Try a different FHR monitor.
- Try a fetal monitor that is not part of a network.
- Use a handheld Doppler ultrasound transducer and hold it in place continuously if needed.

UTERINE ACTIVITY ASSESSMENT

Overview

- Uterine activity should be assessed every time the FHR is assessed.
- Adequate contractions are needed for cervical dilation and effacement to occur.
- Uterine contractions are quantified as the number of contractions present in a 10-minute window, averaged over 30 minutes.
- Characteristics of contractions include:
  - Frequency (how often they occur)
    - Monitor for increased frequency.
    - Too many contractions prevent the fetus from receiving adequate oxygen.
  - Duration (how long they last from beginning to end of the contraction)

(continued)

Overview (continued)

- Strength (how strong they are)
  - ○ Palpation is the most common method of determining strength, but it is subjective.
  - ○ To take a true assessment of strength, insert an IUPC. The cervix must be dilated, and membranes must be ruptured.
- Hormones affect uterine activity:
  - Prior to labor, maternal progesterone levels drop, and estrogen levels rise. The predominance of estrogen increases contractions of the uterus.
- Contractions can be described as normal or abnormal.

Normal Contractions

- Normal: A contraction frequency of one contraction every 2 to 3 minutes (five or fewer contractions in 10 minutes, averaged over a 30-minute window)
- A contraction duration of 60 to 90 seconds
- A contraction strength that is assessed by palpation
  - Strength is assessed as mild, moderate, or strong.
  - Resting tone (uterine tone between contractions) should be soft (or relaxed).

Abnormal Contractions

- Abnormal: Contractions that cannot be characterized as normal frequency, duration, or strength
- Can be characterized as functional dystocia or tachysystole
- Functional dystocia (abnormal, dysfunctional labor):
  - Abnormally slow progress of labor and failure of the cervix to dilate; may be due to:
    - ○ Irregular mild contractions
    - ○ Slow (protracted) or no change in cervical dilatation (arrest of dilatation)
- Tachysystole
  - *Tachysystole*: More than five contractions in 10 minutes, averaged over a 30-minute window
    - ○ Maternal spiral arterioles compressed without adequate relaxation time to perfuse the placenta sufficiently
    - ○ Impairs the transfer of available oxygen to the fetus
  - Can lead to a rising FHR baseline, fewer accelerations, less variability, repetitive decelerations, tachycardia, or bradycardia

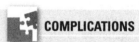 **COMPLICATIONS**

Dysfunctional labor can lead to prolonged labor, increasing the risk for chorioamnionitis. Tachysystole can lead to decreased fetal oxygenation, which can lead to fetal hypoxia. In both instances, the risk of cesarean section is increased.

Causes of Abnormal Contractions

- Causes of functional dystocia
  - Labor induction because labor did not start
  - Large fetus
  - Overdistended uterus from polyhydramnios or multiple gestation

- Causes of tachysystole
  - Medications
    - Adenosine triphosphate
    - Cocaine
    - Prostaglandins
  - Placental abruption
  - Spontaneous labor
  - Uterotonics: Oxytocin

Nursing Interventions

- For dysfunctional labor, administer prostaglandins and/or uterotonics as ordered. Amniotomy may be performed.
- For tachysystole:
  - Administer IV fluid bolus of lactated Ringer's solution.
  - Decrease or discontinue the oxytocin rate.
  - Remove the dinoprostone insert (medication used to prepare cervix).
  - Withhold the next dose of misoprostol.
  - If no response, terbutaline 0.25 mg subcutaneously may be considered.
  - Reposition patient on the right or left side.
  - Administer oxygen, 8 to 10 L per mask.

NURSING PEARL

Resting tone is the pressure exerted by uterine muscle cells when they are at rest between contractions. The strength of resting tone can only be palpated or measured by IUPC. The resting tone should palpate soft or measure 5 to 25 mmHg per IUPC for at least 1 minute to allow the fetus maximum oxygenation between contractions.

POP QUIZ 3.3

A new nurse is learning about contractions and asks how they would know whether their patient is in tachysystole. How would you educate this nurse?

FETAL ASSESSMENT METHODS

Overview

- Assessments can be used to determine fetal well-being with or without fetal monitoring.
- Assessment methods include auscultation, nonstress test, BPP, BPP: modified, CST, fetal movement, umbilical cord blood gas sampling, vibroacoustic stimulation, and fetal scalp stimulation.

Auscultation

Indications
- *Auscultation* is a noninvasive method for low-risk laboring patients that uses the FHR fetoscope, a handheld Doppler ultrasound transducer, or a bedside ultrasound.

Equipment and Procedure
- Fetoscope
  - A fetoscope is a type of stethoscope used to listen to, or auscultate, the FHR.
  - Place the fetoscope on the patient's abdomen to listen for the fetal heartbeat.
  - Count the FHR by using a timer or a watch or clock with a second hand. FHR is calculated in bpm.

(continued)

Equipment and Procedure *(continued)*

- Handheld Doppler ultrasound transducer
  - A handheld Doppler ultrasound transducer is a small device that is placed on the patient's abdomen and displays the FHR. It requires batteries or a plug to charge it.
- Bedside ultrasound
  - Bedside ultrasound allows the person using it to hear the FHR and see an ultrasound picture of the fetal heart.
  - Ultrasounds are expensive and may require batteries or a plug to charge them.
  - 2D or 3D ultrasound is available to produce images of the fetus.

Interpretation of Findings
Fetal heart rate interpretation is discussed in Chapter 4.

Nursing Interventions
- Perform auscultation using available equipment.
- Document FHR assessment.
- Escalate to continuous fetal monitoring if the FHR is not reassuring.
- Check the patient's pulse while checking FHR.

Nonstress Test

Indications
- A nonstress test determines fetal well-being by evaluating fetal oxygenation status and assessing how the FHR responds to fetal movement.
- Antenatal fetal surveillance at 32 0/7 weeks' gestation or later is appropriate for most at-risk or high-risk patients.
- Indications for a nonstress test include:
  - Advanced patient age, history of complications in previous pregnancy (previous fetal demise, underlying fetal conditions), postterm pregnancy, multiple gestation, placental complications, vaginal bleeding or spotting
  - Gestational hypertension, GDM, cholestasis, pre-eclampsia (e.g., headache, visual symptoms), Rh sensitization, sickle-cell anemia, substance abuse
  - Decreased fetal movement, fetal tachycardia, or bradycardia
  - IUGR
  - Oligohydramnios or polyhydramnios, which may cause IUGR

Equipment and Procedure
- Position patient in semi-Fowler's or lateral recumbent position.
- Place ultrasound transducer and tocodynamometer on patient's abdomen.
- Use an external fetal monitor to continuously monitor contractions (if any) and FHR.
- To perform vibroacoustic stimulation, have the patient push the button every time fetal movement is felt.
- Monitor the fetus for 20 to 40 minutes.
- Document fetal assessment.

Interpretation of Findings

- Results of the test may show that the fetus is in a sleep cycle.
- Results may indicate the need for further monitoring and testing or for delivery.
- The findings of a nonstress test are interpreted as either reactive or nonreactive.
  - *Reactive* is considered the normal result (Figure 3.3).
  - Reactive findings include:
    - ○ 32 weeks' or greater gestation: Results are considered reactive if two or more accelerations (at least 15 bpm lasting 15 seconds) occur within a 20-minute period.
    - ○ Less than 32 weeks' gestation: Results are considered reactive if two or more accelerations (at least 10 bpm lasting 10 seconds) occur within a 20-minute period.
    - ○ Accelerations must be achieved within 40 minutes to be considered reactive.
- Nonreactive findings require further testing, possibly including a BPP (see Figure 3.3).

COMPLICATIONS

Oligohydramnios (defined as an amniotic fluid volume of 2 cm or less in the single deepest vertical pocket) should prompt further evaluation even if all other components are normal.

POP QUIZ 3.4

A patient undergoing a nonstress test has been on the monitor for 30 minutes with no accelerations. What could be happening, and what can be done to elicit accelerations?

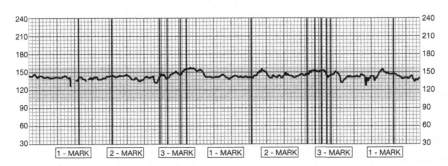

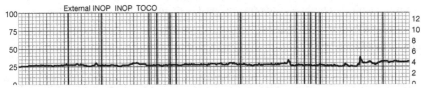

Figure 3.3 An example of a reactive nonstress test.

Source: Nye, R. (2019). *Essentials of fetal heart rate monitoring.* Springer Publishing Company. https://doi .org/10.1891/9780826174246.0006

Nursing Interventions
- Notify provider of results.

Biophysical Profile

Indications
- The BPP consists of a nonstress test based on the FHR monitor and on observations of fetal breathing, movement, tone, and amniotic fluid measurement made by real-time ultrasonography while the patient is lying down.
- The nonstress test may be omitted without compromising test validity if the results of all four ultrasound components of the BPP are within expected ranges.

Equipment and Procedure
- Ultrasound used by the ultrasonographer to determine breathing, movement, tone, and amniotic fluid measurement
- FHR monitor used to assess FHR

Interpretation of Findings
- Expected fetal observations:
  - Fetal breathing: One or more episodes of rhythmic fetal breathing lasting 30 seconds or more within 30 minutes
  - Fetal movement: Three or more discrete body or limb movements within 30 minutes
  - Fetal tone: One or more episodes of extension of a fetal extremity with return to flexion, or opening or closing of a hand
  - Amniotic fluid volume: Amniotic fluid volume greater than 2 cm in the deepest vertical pocket considered evidence of adequate amniotic fluid
- Results: Each of the five components is assigned a score of either 2 (present) or 0 (not present).
  - Normal composite score: 8 or 10
  - Equivocal composite score: 6
  - Abnormal composite score: 4 or less

Nursing Intervention
- If a BPP presents with abnormal results, the patient may be sent to L&D for prolonged fetal monitoring and/or induction of labor.

Biophysical Profile: Modified

Indications
- The modified BPP combines the nonstress test with an amniotic fluid volume assessment performed by ultrasound.

Equipment and Procedure
- FHR monitor used to assess FHR
- Ultrasound used by ultrasonographer or provider to determine amniotic fluid volume

Interpretation of Findings

- Results:
  - Normal: Nonstress test is reactive, and the amniotic fluid volume is greater than 2 cm in the deepest vertical pocket.
  - Abnormal: Nonstress test is nonreactive, or amniotic fluid volume in the deepest vertical pocket is 2 cm or less.

Nursing Interventions

- If a reactive nonstress test is not achieved within 40 minutes, the patient needs additional fetal monitoring.
- If modified BPP presents abnormal results, the patient may be sent to L&D for prolonged fetal monitoring and/or induction of labor.

Contraction Stress Test

Indications

- The CST is ordered for an atypical nonstress test and/or for concerns about fetal well-being and fetal ability to tolerate labor.
  - Fetal well-being is based on the response of the FHR to uterine contractions.
  - Fetal oxygenation will be transiently worsened by uterine contractions.

Equipment and Procedure

- Procedure:
  - Place patient on FHR monitor.
  - Initiate contractions with nipple stimulation or oxytocin.
  - Assess FHR and contraction pattern with continuous EFM.
- Discontinue nipple stimulation or oxytocin when test is complete.
- If prolonged deceleration or bradycardia of FHR is observed, discontinue test immediately.

Interpretation of Findings

- Results are categorized as:
  - Negative: No late or significant variable decelerations
  - Positive: Late decelerations after 50% or more of contractions (even if contraction frequency is fewer than three in 10 minutes)
  - Equivocal–Suspicious: Intermittent late decelerations or significant variable decelerations
  - Equivocal: Decelerations that occur in the presence of contractions more frequently than every 2 minutes or lasting longer than 90 seconds
  - Unsatisfactory: Fewer than three contractions in 10 minutes or an uninterpretable tracing

Nursing Interventions

- Notify provider of results.

 ALERT!

A positive CST may indicate the need for a cesarean section delivery. A patient with abnormal results may be sent to L&D for prolonged fetal monitoring and/or induction of labor.

Fetal Movement

Indications

- May be measured by all pregnant patients in the third trimester to assess fetal well-being.

Equipment and Procedure

- Fetal kick count
  - Fetal kick counts are recommended for all pregnancies after 28 weeks.
  - Instruct patient to move into a side-lying position and to count the number of kicks or fetal movements felt within 2 hours.
    - It is expected and reassuring to feel 10 or more movements within 2 hours.
    - It is discouraging to feel fewer than 10 movements within 2 hours.
- Palpation
  - The patient can palpate the abdomen to feel fetal movement.
  - The nurse or provider can palpate for fetal movement if the patient is unsure of movement.

Interpretation of Findings

- Ten or more movements within 2 hours is normal.
- Fewer than 10 movements may require further monitoring and/or assessment.

Nursing Interventions

- Educate patient about kick counts.
- Nurse should request a nonstress test for high-risk patients if indicated.
- Results:
  - Document fetal assessment.
  - Notify provider of results.

Umbilical Cord Blood Gas Testing

Indications

- Fetal and maternal circulation meets at the placenta, where gas and nutrient exchange occurs.
- The umbilical cord contains three blood vessels:
  - One large vein carrying oxygenated blood to the fetus
  - Two small arteries carrying deoxygenated blood that is relatively rich in carbon dioxide and other metabolic waste products from the fetus
- Oxygen and nutrients diffuse across the placental membrane from maternal arterial blood and are transported to the fetus via the single large UV.
- Fetal blood returns to the placenta following tissue extraction of oxygen and nutrients via the two small UAs.
- The now-deoxygenated blood containing waste products of fetal metabolism (including carbon dioxide) is in maternal circulation and eliminated via maternal lungs and kidneys.
- Sampling umbilical cord gas for an acid–base result provides an objective assessment of fetal metabolic condition at delivery.

- Indications for umbilical cord blood gas testing:
  - Cesarean delivery for fetal compromise
  - Intrapartum fever
  - Apgar less than 7 at 5-minute intervals
  - Maternal thyroid disease
  - Multifetal gestation
  - Severe IUGR
  - Placenta abruption
  - Uterine rupture
  - Fetal and maternal blood loss

 NURSING PEARL

It is important to obtain arterial blood for a cord gas test. When obtaining samples from both types of blood vessels, ensure that one sample is an arterial sample. Arterial cord blood reflects neonatal acid–base status, whereas venous cord blood reflects the combined effect of maternal acid–base status and placental function.

Equipment and Procedure

- Clamp and cut a portion of the umbilical cord.
- Obtain a syringe designated for collection of cord blood gas (per facility policy).
- First, collect arterial blood from UA.
- Next, collect blood from UV.

 ALERT!

Collect blood from the artery before the vein to prevent collapse of the vessels.

Interpretation of Findings

- Metabolic acidosis (reduced blood pH and decreased base) implies that sometime during labor, oxygenation of fetal tissues was severely compromised.

Nursing Interventions

- Table 3.1 shows normal umbilical artery and vein values. Report abnormal results to provider.

Table 3.1 Normal Umbilical Artery and Vein Values

Parameter	Umbilical Artery	Umbilical Vein
pH	7.12–7.35	7.23–7.44
pO_2	6.2–27.6	16.4–40.0
pCO_2	41.9–73.5	28.8–53.3
Bicarbonate	18.8–28.2	17.2–25.6
Base deficit	+9.3 to −1.5	+8.3 to −2.6

Source: Data from Armstrong, L., & Stenson, B. J. (2007). Use of umbilical cord blood gas analysis in the assessment of the newborn. *Archives of Disease in Childhood. Fetal and Neonatal Edition, 92*(6), F430–F434. https://doi.org/10.1136/adc.2006.099846

Vibroacoustic Stimulation

Indications

- Vibroacoustic stimulation consists of vibration and sound applied to the patient's abdomen to elicit a fetal response.
- Indications are:
  - To awaken the fetus during a nonstress test
  - To elicit FHR acceleration indicating reactive fetal status

Equipment and Procedure

- Equipment used is a handheld transducer that delivers an oscillating sound.
- Interpret FHR baseline prior to giving stimulus.
- Perform vibroacoustic stimulation:
  - Maintain continuous FHR tracing.
  - Explain the procedure to the patient.
  - Position the transducer on the patient's abdomen.
  - Apply a stimulus from the transducer for 1 to 2 seconds.
  - Assess the FHR tracing after each stimulus to observe for accelerations.
  - If no response, stimulation may be repeated up to three times for progressively longer durations of up to 3 seconds. If still no response, the results are considered nonreactive.
- Continue to maintain continuous FHR tracing after stimulation.

Interpretation of Findings

- See Figure 3.4.

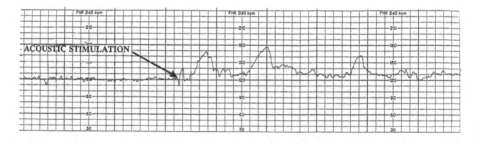
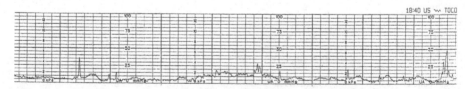

Figure 3.4 FHR showing accelerations after vibroacoustic stimulation.

Source: Murray, M., Huelsmann, G., and Koperski, N. (2019). *Essentials of fetal and uterine monitoring.* Springer Publishing Company.

Nursing Interventions
- Avoid performing vibroacoustic stimulation after a deceleration.
- Notify provider if FHR decelerations are noted or if there is no change in FHR tracing.

Fetal Scalp Stimulation

Indications
- Fetal scalp stimulation is used if the fetal scalp is accessible.
- Fetal scalp stimulation is used when no fetal accelerations are detected on the EFM.
- Gentle rubbing of the fetal scalp may elicit an acceleration to rule out metabolic acidosis.

Equipment and Procedure
- Fetal scalp stimulation may be performed after rupture of membranes if all of the following are true:
  - Cervix is dilated at least 3 cm.
  - Membranes are ruptured.
  - Fetus is engaged at a −1/-2 station.
- Contraindications:
  - Cervix closed
  - Infection
  - Amniotic sac intact or not ruptured
  - Fetal distress noted
- The provider will don a sterile glove and gently touch or rub the fetal scalp for a few seconds to no longer than 15 seconds.

Interpretation of Findings
- An acceleration of the FHR to 15 bpm lasting at least 15 seconds usually reflects a normal fetal scalp pH.
- No acceleration may require interventions based on the FHR.

Nursing Interventions
- Assist the provider at the bedside.
- Assess FHR continuously.
- Assess FHR for accelerations.

 POP QUIZ 3.5

The nurse has difficulty maintaining the FHR tracing on the monitor while the patient is pushing. The FHR is accelerating with contractions. Is this considered normal? What is the next appropriate step?

RESOURCES

American College of Obstetricians and Gynecologists. (2006). American College of Obstetricians and Gynecologists Committee Opinion No. 348, November 2006: Umbilical cord blood gas and acid-base analysis. *Obstetrics & Gynecology, 108*(5), 1319–1322. https://doi .org/10.1097/00006250-200611000-00058

American College of Obstetricians and Gynecologists. (2009). American College of Obstetricians and Gynecologists Practice Bulletin No. 106: Intrapartum fetal heart rate monitoring: Nomenclature, interpretation, and general management principles. *Obstetrics & Gynecology, 114*(1), 192–202. https://doi.org/10.1097/aog.0b013e3181aef106

American College of Obstetricians and Gynecologists. (2014). Obstetric care consensus: Safe prevention of the primary cesarean delivery. *Obstetrics & Gynecology, 123*(3), 693–711. https://doi .org/10.1097/01.aog.0000444441.04111.1d

American College of Obstetricians and Gynecologists. (2020). American College of Obstetricians and Gynecologists Practice Bulletin No. 145: Antepartum fetal surveillance. *Obstetrics & Gynecology, 124,* 182–192. https://doi.org/10.1097/01.AOG.0000451759.90082.7b

Armstrong, L., & Stenson, B. J. (2007). Use of umbilical cord blood gas analysis in the assessment of the newborn. *Archives of Disease in Childhood. Fetal and Neonatal Edition, 92*(6), F430–F434. https://doi.org/10.1136/adc.2006.099846

Association of Women's Health, Obstetric and Neonatal Nurses. (2021). *AWHONN position statements.* https://www.awhonn.org/news-advocacy-and-publications/awhonn-position-stateme nts/

Electronic Fetal Monitoring Basic and Advanced Study. (n.d). *Basic pattern recognition.* http://www .ob-efm.com/efm-basics/basic-pattern-recognition/

Groll, C. G. (2016). *Fast facts for the L&D nurse: labor & delivery orientation in a nutshell.* Springer Publishing Company.

Heelan, L. (2013). Fetal monitoring: creating a culture of safety with informed choice. *Journal of Perinatal Education, 22*(3), 156–165. https://doi.org/10.1891/1058-1243.22.3.156

Kiely, D. J., Oppenheimer, L. W., & Dornan, J. C. (2019). Unrecognized maternal heart rate artefact in cases of perinatal mortality reported to the United States Food and Drug Administration from 2009 to 2019: A critical patient safety issue. *BMC Pregnancy and Childbirth, 19*(1), 501. https://doi .org/10.1186/s12884-019-2660-5. https://pubmed.ncbi.nlm.nih.gov/31842798/

Mdoe, P. F., Ersdal, H. L., Mduma, E., Moshiro, R., Kidanto, H., & Mbekenga, C. (2018). Midwives' perceptions on using a fetoscope and Doppler for fetal heart rate assessments during labor: A qualitative study in rural Tanzania. *BMC Pregnancy Childbirth, 18,* 103. https://doi.org/10.1186/ s12884-018-1736-y

Murray, M., Huelsmann, G., & Koperski, N. (2019). *Essentials of fetal and uterine monitoring.* Springer Publishing Company.

Nye, R. (2019). *Essentials of fetal heart rate monitoring.* Springer Publishing Company. https://doi. org/10.1891/9780826174246.0006

Shakouri, F., Iorizzo, L., Edwards, H. M., Vinter, C. A., Krisensen, K., Isberg, P.-E., & Wiberg, N. (2020). Effectiveness of fetal scalp stimulation test in assessing fetal wellbeing during labor, a retrospective cohort study. *BMC Pregnancy Childbirth, 20,* 347. https://doi.org/10.1186/ s12884-020-03030-7

4

ELECTRONIC FETAL MONITORING PATTERN RECOGNITION

CATEGORIES OF FETAL HEART RATE TRACINGS

Overview

Three categories of FHR tracings are used to classify the health of the fetus while using EFM (Table 4.1).

- Category I: Normal
- Category II: Indeterminate
- Category III: Abnormal

Category I: Normal

- Accelerations present or absent
- Baseline 110 to 160 bpm (see section titled "Fetal Heart Rate Baseline.")
- Baseline variability moderate
- Early decelerations present or absent
- Late or variable decelerations absent
- Strongly predictive of normal fetal acid–base status at the time of observation

Table 4.1 Three Categories of FHR Tracings for Using EFM

Category I	Category II	Category III
All of the following:	*Examples:*	*Either:*

• Baseline 110–160
• Variability:
  • Moderate
• Late or variable decelerations:
  • Absent
• Early decelerations:
  • Present or absent
• Accelerations:
  • Present or absent
	• Moderate variability with recurrent late or variable decelerations
	• Minimal variability with recurrent variable decelerations
	• Absent variability without recurrent decelerations
	• Bradycardia with moderate variability
	• Prolonged decelerations
		• Absent variability with:
		  • Recurrent late decelerations
		  or
		  • Recurrent variable decelerations
		  or
		  • Bradycardia
		  or
		  • Sinusoidal pattern

Source: Nye, R. (2019). *Essentials of fetal heart rate monitoring.* Springer Publishing Company. https://doi.org/10.189 1/9780826174246.0006

Nursing Interventions
- No immediate intervention is needed for a normal FHR.
- Continue to observe FHR per facility policy.
- Document findings.

Category II: Indeterminate

- Any tracing not meeting category I or III criteria:
  - Absence of induced accelerations after fetal stimulation
  - Absent variability without recurrent decelerations
  - Baseline bradycardia not accompanied by absent baseline variability
  - Baseline tachycardia
  - Marked variability
  - Minimal variability
  - Prolonged deceleration
  - Recurrent late decelerations with moderate variability
  - Recurrent variable decelerations with minimal or moderate variability
  - Variable decelerations

Nursing Interventions
- Interventions depend on the characteristics of FHR variability (or lack of variability) and their cause:
  - Administer IV fluid bolus.
  - Administer oxygen: 8-10 L per nonrebreather mask.
  - Discontinue oxytocin (if running).
  - Notify provider.
  - Reposition patient.
- Monitor FHR closely.

 ALERT!

There is evidence to suggest that the longer the FHR remains in category II, especially during the last 2 hours before birth, the greater the risk of neonatal morbidity.

Category III: Abnormal

- Absent variability with any of the following:
  - Bradycardia
  - Recurrent late decelerations
  - Recurrent variable decelerations
- Predictive of abnormal fetal acid–base status at the time of observation
- Sinusoidal pattern

Nursing Interventions
- Notify the provider.
- Prepare for urgent delivery.

FETAL HEART RATE BASELINE

Overview

- Baseline must be determined before the FHR can be categorized.
- Baseline is the mean FHR rounded to 5 bpm during a 10-minute segment.
  - The minimum baseline duration must be at least 2 continuous minutes.
  - This segment must exclude accelerations, decelerations, and periods of marked variability.
- Examples of baseline FHR:
  - Bradycardia: Less than 110 bpm
  - Normal: 110 to 160 bpm
  - Tachycardia: More than160 bpm
- Measure FHR baseline with properly calibrated EFM equipment (wired or wireless).

Influencing Mechanisms of Fetal Heart Rate Baseline

- Common nonphysiological mechanisms that influence FHR baseline:
  - Fetal: Prematurity, sleep cycles
  - Maternal: Medications
- Physiological mechanisms that influence FHR baseline:
  - Fetal: Anemia, cardiac arrhythmias, congenital anomalies, preexisting neurologic conditions
  - Maternal: Hyperthyroidism, interruption of fetal oxygenation, fever, infection, metabolic acidemia

Nursing Interventions

- Determine and treat abnormal baseline if possible.
- Improve transfer of oxygen to the fetus by increasing placental perfusion:
  - Administer IV fluid.
  - Administer supplemental maternal oxygen at 8 to 10 L per nonrebreather mask.
  - Change the patient's position.
  - Prepare for possible emergent delivery, if indicated.

 COMPLICATIONS

Both bradycardia and tachycardia can indicate fetal complications. Prolonged bradycardia of less than 80 bpm for 3 minutes or longer indicates severe hypoxia of the fetus. Persistent tachycardia of greater than 180 bpm, especially occurring in conjunction with maternal fever, suggests chorioamnionitis.

 NURSING PEARL

If minimum baseline duration is less than 2 minutes, then the baseline is indeterminate. For example, if there are prolonged accelerations or repetitive decelerations that do not allow for any 2 continuous minutes of baseline, then the baseline is indeterminate.

 ALERT!

Manage specific FHR patterns per guidelines. Observe and confirm baseline patterns, document changes or trends over time, and document and evaluate fetal response to possible interruption of oxygen pathways and interventions to improve pathways. An abnormal baseline may be acceptable, such as with a premature fetus or a fetus with a known heart condition; a premature fetus may have an abnormally high baseline. Review the entire fetal heart tracing, consider maternal and fetal factors that may affect the tracing, and respond appropriately.

(continued)

Nursing Interventions (continued)
- Monitor and document:
  - Baseline rate and patterns
  - Presence or absence of accelerations and decelerations
  - Interventions and response of the patient and/or fetus
  - Communication with provider
- Monitor FHR baseline concurrently with uterine contractions and document every 15 to 30 minutes.

POP QUIZ 4.1

The nurse is caring for a pregnant patient, and the fetus has a sudden event of bradycardia of 100 bpm, lasting for 4 minutes. What four steps should the nurse take?

FETAL HEART RATE VARIABILITY

Overview
- Classifications (Table 4.2)
  - Absent
  - Minimal
  - Moderate
  - Marked
- Variability is:
  - Fluctuation of the FHR from the baseline in bpm
  - Measured by assessing difference in FHR compared with the baseline of the FHR
- Variability is the most important determinant of fetal well-being.
- Interventions are based on variability compared to the baseline.
- Interventions may also be influenced by the presence or absence of accelerations and/or decelerations, as well as other factors.

COMPLICATIONS

A fetus with persistent minimal or absent variability FHR is at risk for severe fetal compromise related to hypoxia.

Table 4.2 Classifications of FHR Variability	
Classification	**Definition**
Absent	Undetectable amplitude range
Minimal	Amplitude range of 1–5 bpm
Moderate	Amplitude range of 6–25 bpm
Marked	Amplitude range of greater than 25 bpm

Absent and Minimal Variability

- Absent variability has an undetectable amplitude range of the FHR (Figure 4.1).
- Absent variability may be a sign of fetal distress.
- Minimal variability has an amplitude range of 1 to 5 bpm (Figure 4.2).
- Minimal variability may suggest opioid administration to the patient, a fetal sleep cycle, or a premature fetus, or it may be a sign of fetal distress.

Causes

- Fetal arrhythmias and congenital anomalies
- Fetal hypoxemia/acidosis
- Fetal sleep cycles
- Fetal tachycardia
- Maternal medications
  - Anesthetics
  - Barbiturates
  - Narcotics: Para-sympatholytics, anesthetics, or similar
  - Phenothiazines
  - Tranquilizers
- Preexisting fetal neurological abnormality
- Prematurity

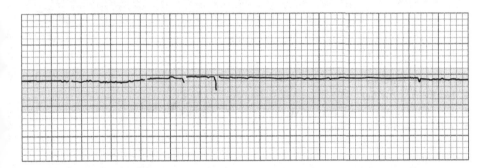

1950 external INOP INOP TOCO

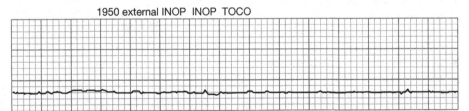

Figure 4.1 Absent variability. This tracing shows smooth fetal heartbeat. It is not possible to determine baseline FHR. This is a category II FHR, which requires close monitoring. (Each small square = 10 seconds; each large square = 1 minute.)

Source: Nye, R. (2019). *Essentials of fetal heart rate monitoring.* Springer Publishing Company. https://doi.org/10.1891/9780826174246.0006

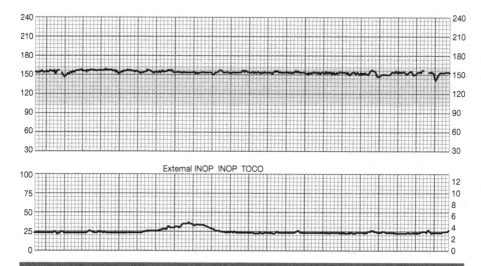

Figure 4.2 Minimal variability with a baseline of 150 bpm. This tracing shows some variability (less than 5 bpm) with no accelerations or decelerations. This is a category II FHR and is concerning. It may indicate a fetal sleep cycle or occur after maternal narcotic administration, but if it persists, it requires intervention. (Each small square = 10 seconds; each large square = 1 minutes.)

Source: Nye, R. (2019). *Essentials of fetal heart rate monitoring* (Figure 3.6). Springer Publishing Company. https://doi.org/10.1891/9780826174246.0006

Nursing Interventions

- Notify the provider.
- Discontinue oxytocin if applicable.
- Administer IV fluid bolus.
- Reposition the patient.
- Determine cause.
- Prepare for operative vaginal birth or cesarean section.
- Administer oxygen 8 to 10 L per nonrebreather mask.
- Document all interventions performed.
- Monitor FHR.
- Evaluate fetal response to interventions.

> **ALERT!**
>
> If a patient is admitted to the labor and delivery unit and the initial FHR variability is minimal to absent, the nurse should urgently alert the provider due to the unknown duration of the nonreassuring pattern. The nurse should continue to monitor.

Moderate Variability

- Has an amplitude range of 6 to 25 bpm
- Signifies the absence of fetal acidosis (Figure 4.3)
- Is reflective of normal variability for a well-oxygenated fetus

Causes

- Nonacidotic fetus (normal)

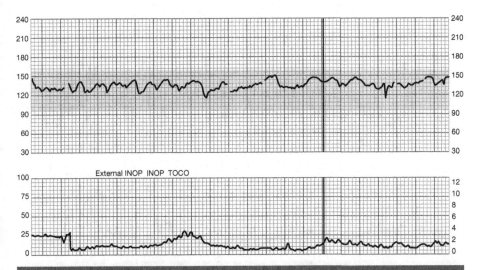

Figure 4.3 Moderate variability with a baseline of 135 bpm. There are accelerations with a peak of 15 bpm, lasting for 15 seconds or more. There are no decelerations. (Each small square = 10 seconds; each large square = 1 minute.) This is a normal, category I FHR that demonstrates a nonacidotic fetus. This FHR does not require any intervention other than observation and documentation of findings.

Source: Nye, R. (2019). *Essentials of fetal heart rate monitoring.* Springer Publishing Company. https://doi. org/10.1891/9780826174246.0006

Nursing Interventions

- Document FHR interpretation per facility policy.
- Monitor FHR per facility policy, as no immediate interventions are needed.

Marked Variability

- Has an amplitude range of greater than 25 bpm (Figure 4.4)
- Is not related to neonatal morbidity, although it has been correlated with abnormal arterial cord blood gases

Causes

- Fetal stimulation:
  - Contractions
  - Vaginal examination
- Maternal medications:
  - Albuterol
  - Terbutaline

 NURSING PEARL

Moderate variability reliably predicts the absence of fetal metabolic acidosis at the time it is observed.

(continued)

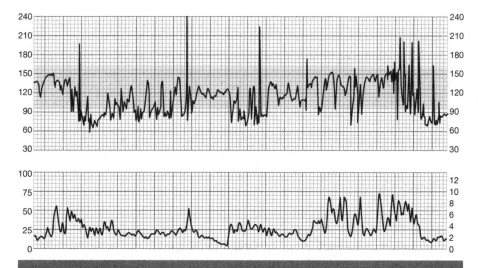

Figure 4.4 Marked variability. The FHR is greater than 25 bpm, making it impossible to determine the baseline or determine accelerations or decelerations. (Each small square = 10 seconds; each large square = 1 minute.) This is a category II FHR that needs further monitoring and notification of provider.

Source: Nye, R. (2019). *Essentials of fetal heart rate monitoring.* Springer Publishing Company. https://doi.org/10.1891/9780826174246.0006

Causes (continued)
- Maternal substances:
  - Cocaine
  - Methamphetamine
  - Nicotine
- Mild hypoxemia

Nursing Interventions
In order of priority:
- Notify the provider.
- Monitor the patient closely.
- Apply an FSE for more accurate reading of FHR variability.
- Determine the cause.
- Document all interventions performed.
- Monitor FHR.
- Evaluate fetal response to interventions.

 POP QUIZ 4.2

What is the most important characteristic of fetal heart tracings in determining fetal well-being?

FETAL HEART RATE ACCELERATIONS

Overview

- Adequate accelerations are:
  - Less than 32 weeks' gestation: Greater than or equal to 10 bpm above baseline for greater than or equal to 10 seconds

- Greater than 32 weeks' gestation: Greater than or equal to 15 bpm above baseline for greater than or equal to 15 seconds
- An *FHR acceleration* is an abrupt increase from FHR baseline with time of onset to peak of acceleration less than 30 seconds, lasting less than 2 minutes (Figure 4.5).
- A *prolonged acceleration* is an increase in heart rate that lasts longer than 2 minutes but less than 10 minutes.

NURSING PEARL

Any acceleration or deceleration that lasts longer than 10 minutes is considered a change in FHR baseline.

Causes

There are many possible causes of FHR acceleration, which may include:
- Fetal movement
- Vaginal examinations
- Uterine contractions
- Umbilical vein compression
- Fetal scalp stimulation
- External acoustic stimulation

Nursing Interventions

- This is a normal, reactive pattern.
- Monitor FHR per facility policy, as no immediate interventions are needed.

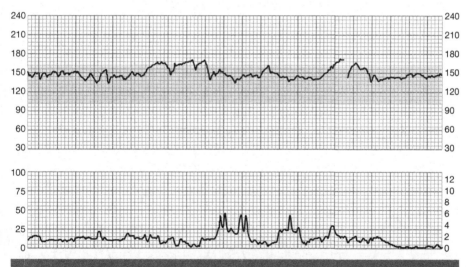

Figure 4.5 FHR showing accelerations. The FHR baseline is 145 bpm with moderate variability. There are accelerations that are at least 15 bpm above baseline and last for at least 15 seconds. There are no decelerations. (Each small square = 10 seconds; each large square = 1 minute.) This is a category I FHR.

Source: Nye, R. (2019). *Essentials of fetal heart rate monitoring.* Springer Publishing Company. https://doi.org/10.1891/9780826174246.0006

FETAL HEART RATE DECELERATIONS

Overview

- Decelerations are:
  - A decrease of FHR below baseline
  - Considered *intermittent* if they occur with less than 50% of contractions in a 20-minute period
  - Considered *recurrent* if they occur with more than 50% of contractions in a 20-minute period
- Types of decelerations are:
  - Early decelerations
  - Late decelerations
  - Periodic or episodic decelerations
  - Prolonged decelerations
  - Variable decelerations

Early Decelerations

- Are gradual decreases in FHR and may be observed as labor progresses.
- Measure more than 30 seconds from onset of deceleration to nadir (the lowest point of a deceleration; occurs with the peak of a contraction; Figure 4.6).

 ALERT!

Early decelerations are not usually seen in early labor. If they are observed in early labor, it could be due to breech presentation. Verify fetal position by vaginal examination or ultrasound.

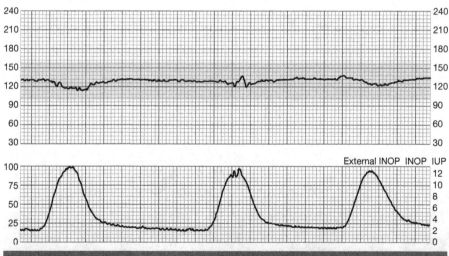

Figure 4.6 Early decelerations observed, mirroring contractions. The FHR baseline is 130 bpm, with minimal variability. There are no accelerations or decelerations. (Each small square = 10 seconds; each large square = 1 minute.) The tracing is category II because of the variability. The decelerations are a normal finding.

Source: Nye, R. (2019). *Essentials of fetal heart rate monitoring.* Springer Publishing Company. https://doi.org/10.1891/9780826174246.0006

- May be observed as labor progresses.
- Are not associated with adverse outcomes.

Causes
- Breech presentation
- Fetal head compression (Figure 4.7)
- Thought to represent a fetal autonomic response to changes in intracranial pressure and/or cerebral blood flow caused by compression of the fetal head during uterine contractions

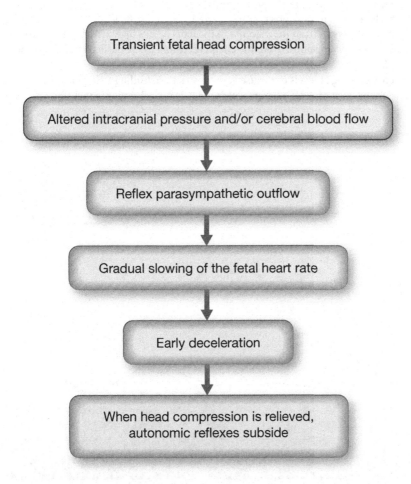

Figure 4.7 Pathophysiology of early deceleration. Fetal head compression triggers blood flow, which triggers the parasympathetic reflex, slowing the FHR.

Source: Nye, R. (2019). *Essentials of fetal heart rate monitoring.* Springer Publishing Company. https://doi.org/10.1891/9780826174246.0006

Nursing Interventions
- Monitor FHR per facility policy, as no immediate interventions are needed. These are normal decelerations.

Late Decelerations

- Late decelerations are a gradual decrease in FHR with onset of deceleration to nadir greater than 30 seconds (Figure 4.8).
- Onset of the deceleration occurs after the beginning of the contraction, and the nadir of the contraction occurs after the peak of the contraction.
- Late deceleration is usually preceded by uteroplacental insufficiency.
  - Decreased oxygen from the placenta to the fetus causes hypoxemia in the fetus, which triggers a response from the chemoreceptors to the baroreceptors, leading to a parasympathetic response and a late deceleration (Figure 4.9).
  - Decreased oxygen levels can cause vasoconstriction, leading to hypertension.
  - Hypertension stimulates a baroreceptor-mediated vagal response that slows the FHR.

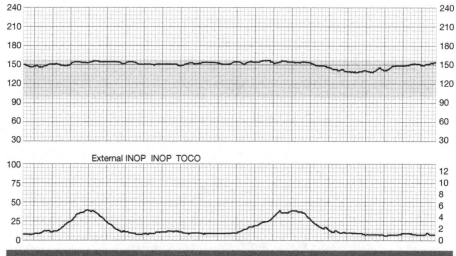

Figure 4.8 Late decelerations. The deceleration begins with the contraction and ends after the contraction finishes, making it a late deceleration. The FHR baseline is 150 bpm with minimal variability. (Each small square = 10 seconds; each large square = 1 minute.) This is a category II FHR, which requires interventions.

Source: Nye, R. (2019). *Essentials of fetal heart rate monitoring.* Springer Publishing Company. https://doi .org/10.1891/9780826174246.0006

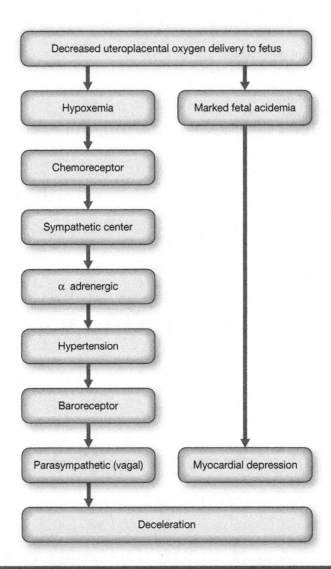

Figure 4.9 Pathophysiology of a late deceleration. Decreased oxygen from the placenta to the fetus causes hypoxemia, which triggers a response from the chemoreceptors to the baroreceptors, leading to a parasympathetic response and a late deceleration. If the placenta does not deliver oxygen to the fetus for a prolonged period, acidemia can occur, leading to myocardial depression and late decelerations.

Source: Nye, R. (2019). *Essentials of fetal heart rate monitoring.* Springer Publishing Company. https://doi.org/10.1891/9780826174246.0006

Causes
- Diabetes
- Excessive uterine contractions
- Fetal IUGR
- Hypertensive disorders
- Maternal hypotension
- Maternal hypoxemia
- Placental abruption

Nursing Interventions
- Administer IV hydration.
- Administer oxygen.
- Correct any hypotension with IV fluid bolus, medications, and/or blood products.
- Discontinue oxytocin.
- Place patient in the lateral position.
- Notify provider if late deceleration persists.

Variable Decelerations

- *Variable deceleration* is a visually apparent, abrupt decrease in FHR.
  - Onset of deceleration to nadir is less than 30 seconds.
  - Heart rate is at least 15 bpm below baseline, lasting between 15 seconds and 2 minutes (Figure 4.10).
- Pathophysiology of variable decelerations (Figure 4.11):

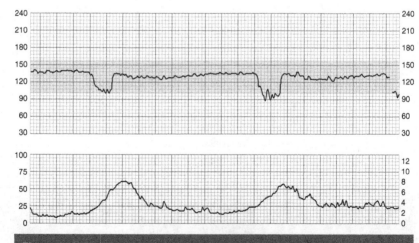

Figure 4.10 Variable decelerations observed. The baseline is 135 bpm. The FHR shows moderate variability with no accelerations and variable decelerations. (Each small square = 10 seconds; each large square = 1 minute.) This is a category II FHR.

Source: Nye, R. (2019). *Essentials of fetal heart rate monitoring.* Springer Publishing Company. https://doi.org/10.1891/9780826174246.0006

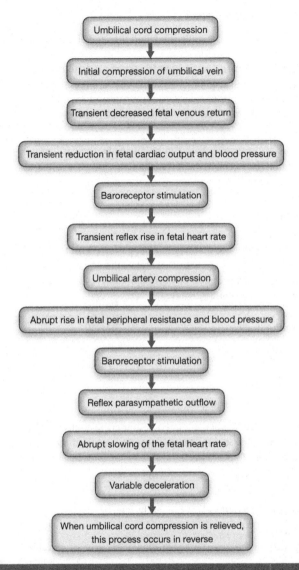

Figure 4.11 Pathophysiology of a variable deceleration. Umbilical cord compression compresses the umbilical vein, leading to decreased venous return, which can trigger baroreceptor stimulation and a transient rise in the FHR. This can be seen as a rise in baseline right before the deceleration, which occurs when the artery is compressed, causing a rise in peripheral resistance. This then causes baroreceptor stimulation, which leads to parasympathetic reflux and an abrupt slowing of the FHR.

Source: Nye, R. (2019). *Essentials of fetal heart rate monitoring.* Springer Publishing Company. https://doi.org/10.1891/9780826174246.0006

(continued)

Variable Decelerations (*continued*)

- Variable decelerations are vagally mediated through chemoreceptors or baroreceptors.
- Decreased venous return causes a baroreceptor-mediated acceleration and decreased arterial oxygen tension secondary to complete cord compression.
- In a premature fetus, variable decelerations can occur with head compression secondary to vagal nerve activation from fetal movement.

Causes
- Umbilical cord compression, which can be caused by the cord wrapping around the fetus's body or neck (also called *nuchal cord*)
- Fetal pressure on umbilical cord
- Prolapsed umbilical cord

Nursing Interventions
- Administer oxygen.
- Change position of patient to rest where FHR pattern is most improved. The Trendelenburg position (supine with feet higher than head) may be helpful.
- Assess for umbilical cord prolapse or imminent delivery with vaginal examination. Umbilical cord prolapse requires emergent cesarean section.
- Prepare for amnioinfusion.
- Discontinue oxytocin.
- Modify patient's pushing to every second or third contraction.

> **POP QUIZ 4.3**
>
> Which type of deceleration would most likely be alleviated with amnioinfusion?

Periodic or Episodic Decelerations

- *Episodic patterns* are those not associated with uterine contractions.
- *Periodic patterns* are those associated with uterine contractions.
- Early and late decelerations are periodic.
- Variable decelerations can be periodic or episodic.

Causes
Cause depends on the type of deceleration: early, late, or variable.

Nursing Interventions
Intervention depends on the type of deceleration: early, late, or variable.

Prolonged Decelerations

- A *prolonged deceleration* is a decrease in FHR of greater than 15 bpm, measured from the most recently determined baseline rate.
- A prolonged deceleration lasts at least 2 minutes but less than 10 minutes (Figure 4.12).

Causes

- Artifact
- Umbilical cord compression
- Umbilical cord prolapse
- Maternal hypotension
- Maternal seizure
- Placental abruption
- Uterine hyperactivity
- Uterine rupture

 NURSING PEARL

VEAL CHOP is a mnemonic used to help remember fetal heart rate patterns (VEAL) and their causes (CHOP):

- Heart Rate Pattern
  - **V**ariable decelerations
  - **E**arly decelerations
  - **A**ccelerations
  - **L**ate decelerations
- Cause
  - **C**ord compression
  - **H**ead compression
  - **O**kay
  - **P**lacental insufficiency

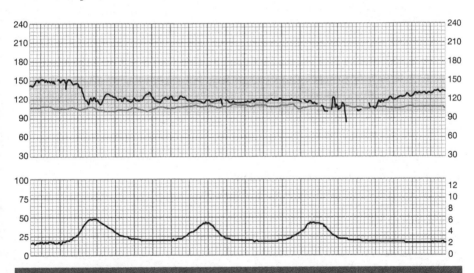

Figure 4.12 A prolonged deceleration lasting approximately 6 minutes. The baseline cannot be determined because 2 minutes of baseline are not shown here. There is minimal to moderate variability and no accelerations. (Each small square = 10 seconds; each large square = 1 minute.) This is a category II FHR that requires interventions.

Source: Nye, R. (2019). *Essentials of fetal heart rate monitoring.* Springer Publishing Company. https://doi.org/10.1891/9780826174246.0006

Nursing Interventions
- Administer IV hydration.
- Administer oxygen.
- Correct any hypotension with IV fluid bolus of normal saline or lactated Ringer's solution, medication, and/or blood products.
- Discontinue oxytocin.
- Place patient in the lateral position.

FETAL ARRYTHMIAS

Overview

- Arrhythmias are classified as:
  - Bradycardia
  - Tachycardia
  - Pseudo-sinusoidal
  - Sinusoidal
- *Fetal arrhythmias* are abnormalities in the FHR baseline that last longer than 10 minutes.
- If an arrhythmia is observed during intermittent fetal monitoring, the patient should be placed on continuous monitoring, and the nurse should assess every 15 minutes or per institutional policy.

Bradycardia

- *Bradycardia* refers to FHR less than 110 bpm in a term fetus or less than 120 bpm in a preterm fetus, lasting longer than 10 minutes.
- Some fetuses have a naturally low baseline FHR, but low-baseline FHR can indicate complications in other cases (Figure 4.13).

Causes
- Asphyxia
- Fetal heart block
- Hypoxia with or without metabolic acidosis
- Maternal hypotension (e.g., after epidural placement)
- Metabolic acidosis
- Placental abruption
- Rapid fetal descent
- Tachysystole
- Umbilical cord prolapse
- Uterine rupture

Nursing Interventions
- Increase fetal perfusion and oxygenation:
  - Administer oxygen.
  - Discontinue oxytocin.
  - Start IV hydration (normal saline or lactated Ringer's solution).

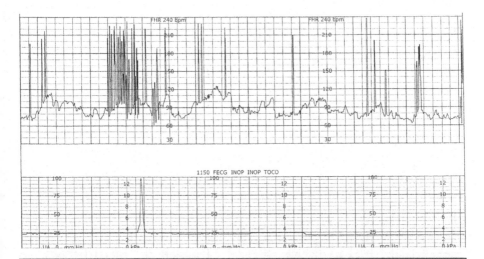

Figure 4.13 FHR showing bradycardia with a baseline FHR of approximately 85 bpm to 90 bpm. (Each small square = 10 seconds; each large square = 1 minute). There is moderate variability and accelerations. This is a category III FHR that requires immediate attention.

Source: Murray, M., Huelsmann, G., and Koperski, N. (2019). *Essentials of fetal and uterine monitoring.* Springer Publishing Company. https://doi.org/10.1891/9780826174246.0006

- Notify provider of new-onset bradycardia. Prepare for an emergency cesarean section if vaginal delivery is not expected in the next few minutes.
- Place patient in lateral position.

Tachycardia

- *Tachycardia* is defined as FHR greater than 160 bpm lasting longer than 10 minutes (Figure 4.14).
  - Tachycardia can be related to vagal suppression and/or sympathetic dominance.

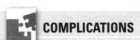 **COMPLICATIONS**

Tachycardia without accelerations but with decreased baseline variability has been demonstrated to cause fetal hypoxia, hypercarbia, and metabolic acidosis.

Causes
- Chorioamnionitis
- Fetal anemia
- Fetal hypoxia
- Fetal tachyarrhythmia
- Fetal heart failure
- Maternal fever
- Medications:
  - Beta sympathomimetics
  - Hydroxyzine pamoate

(continued)

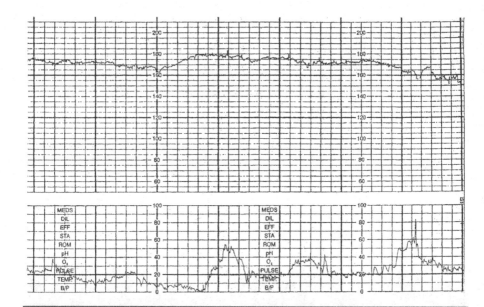

Figure 4.14 FHR showing tachycardia with a baseline FHR of approximately 170 bpm. The variability is moderate, with accelerations and no decelerations, although the end of the tracing may be the beginning of a deceleration. (Each small square = 10 seconds; each large square = 1 minute.) This is a category II FHR tracing, which requires interventions.

Source: Murray, M., Huelsmann, G., & Koperski, N. (2019). *Essentials of fetal and uterine monitoring.* Springer Publishing Company.

Causes (continued)
- Phenothiazines
- Tocolytic: terbutaline

Nursing Interventions
- Assess patient to evaluate and treat cause of fetal tachycardia.
- Notify provider.
- Treat patient fever and infection per provider orders.

 NURSING PEARL

Maternal fever is the most common cause of new-onset fetal tachycardia.

Pseudo-Sinusoidal

- *Pseudo-sinusoidal* is a smooth, wave-like, undulating pattern with a cycle frequency of 3 to 5 minutes.
- It is characterized by fluctuations in the baseline that are regular in amplitude and frequency.
- Pattern stops after 30 to 40 minutes.

Causes
- Fetal sleep cycle
- Maternal narcotics

Nursing Interventions

- Monitor for at least 20 minutes:
  - If the patient received narcotics
  - To determine whether the cause of pattern is a fetal sleep cycle
- Notify the provider if pattern persists.

Sinusoidal

- *Sinusoidal* is a smooth, wave-like, undulating pattern with a cycle frequency of 3 to 5 minutes persisting for at least 20 minutes (Figure 4.15).
- It is characterized by fluctuations in the baseline, which are regular in amplitude and frequency.
- A sinusoidal pattern is an ominous FHR pattern associated with neonatal morbidity and mortality.

Causes

- Fetal hypoxia
- Severe fetal anemia, such as abruption or ABO incompatibility

Nursing Interventions

- Prepare for emergent delivery, to include cesarean section if vaginal delivery is not imminent.

 ALERT!

It is important for the nurse to determine the cause for a pseudo-sinusoidal pattern by looking at the overall tracing for longer than 20 minutes. Narcotic administration and fetal sleep cycles can cause a pseudo-sinusoidal pattern. Consider risk factors for a sinusoidal pattern, and, if the nurse is unsure of the cause, notify the provider.

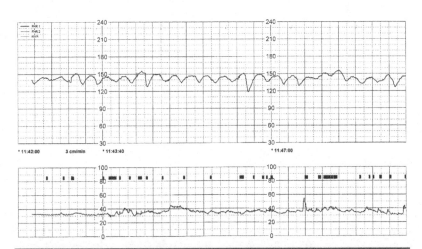

Figure 4.15 A sinusoidal pattern. (Each small square = 10 seconds; each large square = 1 minute.) The baseline of this FHR is approximately 140 bpm. The variability is not determined in a sinusoidal pattern. There are no accelerations or decelerations. This is a category III FHR, which requires immediate interventions.

Source: Murray, M., Huelsmann, G., & Koperski, N. (2019). *Essentials of fetal and uterine monitoring.* Springer Publishing Company.

RESOURCES

American College of Obstetricians and Gynecologists. (2015). Practice bulletin No. 116: Management of intrapartum fetal heart rate tracings. *Obstetrics & Gynecology, 116*(5), 1232–1240. https://doi.org/ 10.1097/AOG.0b013e3182004fa9. https://journals.lww.com/greenjournal/Citation/2010/11000/ Practice_Bulletin_No__116__Management_of.53.aspx

Association of Women's Health, Obstetric and Neonatal Nurses. (2015). *Fetal heart monitoring: Principles and practices (AWHONN, Fetal Heart Monitoring)* (5th ed.). Kendall Hunt Publishing Company.

Cahill, A. G., & Spain, J. (2015). Intrapartum fetal monitoring. *Clinical Obstetrics and Gynecology, 58*(2), 263–268. https://doi.org/10.1097/GRF.0000000000000

Miller, L. A., Miller, D. A., & Cypher, R. L. (2017). *Mosby's pocket guide to fetal monitoring: a multidisciplinary approach*. Elsevier.

Murray, M., Huelsmann, G., & Koperski, N. (2019). *Essentials of fetal and uterine monitoring*. Springer Publishing Company.

National Certification Corporation. (2016). *2016 NCC monograph free version.pdf.* https://ncc-efm. org/filz/2016%20NCC%20Monograph%20Free%20Version.pdf

Nye, R. (2019). *Essentials of fetal heart rate monitoring*. Springer Publishing Company. https://doi. org/10.1891/9780826174246.0006

Polnaszek, B., López, J. D., Clark, R., Raghuraman, N., Macones, G. A., & Cahill, A. G. (2020). Marked variability in intrapartum electronic fetal heart rate patterns: Association with neonatal morbidity and abnormal arterial cord gas. *Journal of Perinatology: Official Journal of the California Perinatal Association, 40*(1), 56–62. https://doi.org/10.1038/s41372-019-0520-9109

Sweha, A., Hacker, T. W., & Nuovo, J. (1999). *Interpretation of the electronic fetal heart rate during labor. American Family Physician, 59*(9), 2487–2500.

5

COMPLICATIONS

FETAL COMPLICATIONS

- In this chapter, fetal complications are partially organized using the categories from Table 2.1 (see Chapter 2):
  - Environmental conditions
  - Maternal respiratory system
  - Maternal blood flow
  - Maternal seizure
  - Uterus
  - Placenta
  - Umbilical cord
  - Fetus
  - Other maternal complications
  - Complications of labor

 ALERT!

All fetal complications can lead to fetal demise if not treated immediately.

ENVIRONMENTAL CONDITIONS

- Pollution
- Smoke (can include particulate matter from fires, air pollution, and secondhand smoke from tobacco products)

Nursing Interventions

- Assess patient via continuous EFM to observe and identify fetal response to any disruption of the maternal–fetal oxygen pathway.
- Implement nursing interventions to increase blood flow to improve uteroplacental circulation and promote fetal oxygenation:
  - Reposition patient to a lateral position.
  - Administer IV fluid bolus.
  - Administer supplemental oxygen:
    - Administer 10 L/min via nonrebreather face mask.
    - Discontinue as soon as possible based on fetal status.
  - Modification of pushing efforts:
    - Pushing with every other or every third contraction
    - Temporary discontinuation of pushing (during second-stage labor)

(continued)

Nursing Interventions *(continued)*

- Decrease oxytocin rate (any or all of the following as indicated):
  - ○ Discontinue oxytocin per order.
  - ○ Remove prostaglandin E2 insert.
  - ○ Withhold next dose of misoprostol.

MATERNAL RESPIRATORY SYSTEM

MATERNAL LUNGS

- Respiratory depression affects the maternal lungs in the maternal–fetal oxygen pathway.
- *Respiratory depression* is defined as slow and ineffective breathing.
- Symptoms of respiratory depression include feeling tired and short of breath.
- Causes of respiratory depression include:
  - Chronic lung diseases such as asthma and cystic fibrosis
  - Hypoventilation
  - Neuromuscular disease
  - Obstructive sleep apnea
- Abnormal maternal respiratory findings can affect fetal oxygenation because they can cause impaired gas exchange.

Nursing Interventions

- Maintain continuous FHR tracing.
- Determine cause of respiratory depression and treat underlying cause.
- Monitor pulse oximetry, respiratory rate, and respiratory status.
- Auscultate breath sounds to determine whether lungs are clear bilaterally.
- Administer supplemental oxygen.
- Administer medication as ordered to improve lung function and gas exchange.

MATERNAL BLOOD FLOW

MATERNAL CARDIAC DISEASE AND BLOOD DISORDERS

- Blood disorders include anemia, sickle cell anemia, and thalassemia.
- Cardiac disease includes congestive heart failure, cardiomyopathy, heart rhythm disorders, heart valve disorders, and congenital heart disease.
- Interruptions to maternal blood flow due to preexisting or chronic conditions can cause decreased cardiac output, which can lead to decreased oxygen in the maternal blood, which then causes decreased oxygenation of the fetus.

Nursing Interventions

- Assess patient via continuous EFM to observe and identify fetal response to any disruption of the maternal–fetal oxygen pathway.
- Implement nursing interventions to increase blood flow and promote fetal oxygenation:
  - Reposition patient into a lateral position.
  - Administer IV fluid bolus.
  - Administer supplemental oxygen:

- ○ Administer 10 L/min via nonrebreather face mask.
- ○ Discontinue as soon as possible based on fetal status.
- Modify pushing efforts.
  - ○ Push with every other or every third contraction
  - ○ Temporary discontinuation of pushing (during second stage labor)
- Decrease oxytocin rate (any or all of the following as indicated):
  - ○ Discontinue oxytocin per order.
  - ○ Remove prostaglandin E2 insert.
  - ○ Withhold next dose of misoprostol.

POP QUIZ 5.1

A 29-year-old patient is 38 weeks' pregnant and has cardiomyopathy. Where in the oxygen pathway is the area of concern for maternal–fetal oxygenation?

MATERNAL HYPOTENSION

- *Hypotension* is typically defined as maternal BP of less than or equal to 90/60 mmHg.
- Causes of maternal hypotension include:
  - Cardiac condition
  - Dehydration
  - Epidural or spinal anesthesia
  - Excessive blood loss, hemorrhage, or hemorrhagic shock
  - Supine position or IVC syndrome
- Hypotension interrupts the maternal–fetal oxygen pathway by reducing placental blood flow, perfusion, and exchange of gases.
- Anesthesia:
  - Epidural or spinal anesthesia affects the nerve fibers that control muscle contractions inside the blood vessels, which causes the blood vessels to relax due to vasodilation, thereby lowering BP. The resulting hypotension can affect fetal oxygenation.
    - ○ Epidural anesthesia is given in labor for pain relief and can be used for an unplanned cesarean section after failure to progress in labor or category III FHR tracing/emergent surgical delivery.
    - ○ Spinal anesthesia is usually given prior to cesarean section.

Nursing Interventions

- Call for additional assistance and notify provider.
- Maintain continuous monitoring of FHR tracing. The nurse may observe:
  - Late decelerations
  - Minimal or absent variability
- Monitor maternal BP.
- Monitor patients with underlying heart conditions with continuous three-lead EKG.
- Reposition patient into left lateral position to increase blood flow back to uterus.
- Administer IV fluid bolus per order. May obtain additional IV access for blood administration if needed.
- Administer supplemental oxygen:
  - Administer 10 L/min via nonrebreather face mask.
  - Discontinue as soon as possible based on fetal status.

(continued)

Nursing Interventions *(continued)*

- Anesthesia-specific nursing interventions:
  - Epidural:
    - ○ Notify provider and anesthesiologist of maternal hypotension and vital signs.
    - ○ Anesthesiologist may administer ephedrine.
  - Spinal: Anesthesia team will manage hypotension in the operating room.

HYPERTENSIVE DISORDERS IN PREGNANCY

- Hypertensive disorders in pregnancy include disorders related to hypertension.
- Hypertensive disorders can be classified as:
  - Chronic hypertension (not pregnancy related)
  - Eclampsia
  - Gestational hypertension
  - HELLP syndrome
  - Preeclampsia: Superimposed, with or without severe features
- *Chronic hypertension* is defined as BP greater than or equal to 140 mmHg systolic and/or 90 mmHg diastolic before pregnancy or before 20 weeks of gestation.

 COMPLICATIONS

Complications for the fetus include fetal growth restriction and preterm birth. Complications to maternal body systems include cardiovascular effects, eclampsia, HELLP syndrome, liver damage, renal damage, retinal damage, placental abruption, pulmonary edema, and neurological effects such as hypertensive encephalopathy. In addition, stroke is the leading cause of maternal morbidity from preeclampsia.

- *Eclampsia* is defined by new-onset tonic-clonic, focal, or multifocal seizures in the absence of other causative conditions.
- *Gestational hypertension* is characterized by systolic BP of 140 mmHg or more or diastolic BP of 90 mmHg or more, or both, on two occasions at least 4 hours apart after 20 weeks of gestation.
- *HELLP syndrome* is diagnosed in patients with *h*emolysis, *e*levated *l*iver enzymes, and *l*ow *p*latelet count.
- *Preeclampsia* is associated with new-onset hypertension, which occurs most often after 20 weeks of gestation and often near term.
  - Preeclampsia is often accompanied by new-onset proteinuria.
  - Preeclampsia is often diagnosed with gestational hypertension and proteinuria (greater than or equal to 300 mg in 24-hour collection or a protein/creatinine ratio of greater than or equal to 0.3 mg/dL).
  - Hypertension and other signs or symptoms of preeclampsia may present in some patients without proteinuria.
- *Gestational hypertension* in the absence of proteinuria is diagnosed with preeclampsia with severe features if any of the following are present:
  - Impaired liver function
  - New-onset headache
  - Pulmonary edema
  - Renal insufficiency

 POP QUIZ 5.2

What is a possible diagnosis for a patient with new onset of seizures during pregnancy or the postpartum period without a preexisting neurologic disorder?

- Severe persistent right upper quadrant or epigastric pain
- Severe range BPs with one of the following:
  - Systolic BP of 160 mmHg or higher
  - Diastolic BP of 110 mmHg or higher
- Thrombocytopenia (platelet count less than 100,000)
- Visual disturbances
- Treatments include:
  - Magnesium sulfate to prevent seizures
  - Medications for severe range BPs
    (Table 5.1):
    - Hydralazine IVP
    - Labetalol IVP
    - Nifedipine immediate-release PO

Causes

- May be indeterminate
- Possible risk factors:
  - Antiphospholipid antibody syndrome
  - Assisted reproductive technology

 NURSING PEARL

Preeclampsia with severe features can cause pulmonary edema. Patients in labor sometimes receive large amounts of IV fluids. It is important to limit fluids for these patients to a total of 125 mL/hr (3,000 mL in 24 hours).

Table 5.1 Medications for Hypertension

Indications	Mechanism of Action	Contraindications, Precautions, and Adverse Effects
Anticonvulsant (magnesium sulfate)		
• Preeclampsia with severe features	• Relaxes smooth muscles to reduce chance of seizures	• Medication is contraindicated in patients with myasthenia gravis. • Side effects include flushing, nausea, diaphoresis, loss of deep tendon reflexes, respiratory depression, and cardiac arrest.
Antidotes (calcium gluconate)		
• Magnesium toxicity	• Direct antagonism of magnesium at the site of action	• There are no contraindications. • Administer slowly through IV push. • Side effects include syncope and bradycardia.
Beta-blockers (labetalol)		
• Hypertensive disorder	• Relax blood vessels and slow heart rate	• Medication is contraindicated in patients with asthma, AV heart block, and hypotension. • Side effects include lightheadedness, shortness of breath, low heart rate, and severe headache.

(continued)

Table 5.1 Medications for Hypertension *(continued)*

Indications	Mechanism of Action	Contraindications, Precautions, and Adverse Effects
Calcium channel blockers (nifedipine)		
• Hypertensive disorder	• Relax muscles in heart	• Medication is contraindicated with hypotension and cardiac lesions.
		• Side effects include flushing, dizziness, hypotension, and slower heart rate.
Vasodilator (hydralazine)		
• Hypertensive disorder	• Relaxes muscles in blood vessels to help them dilate	• Medication is contraindicated in patients with coronary artery disease or rheumatic heart disease affecting the mitral valve.
		• Side effects include chest pain or pressure, light-headed feeling, and numbness in hands and feet.

Causes *(continued)*

- Chronic hypertension
- Gestational diabetes
- Maternal age 35 years or older
- Multifetal gestations
- Nulliparity
- Obstructive sleep apnea
- Preeclampsia in a previous pregnancy
- Pregestational diabetes
- Prepregnancy BMI greater than 30
- Renal disease
- Systemic lupus erythematosus
- Thrombophilia

Nursing Interventions

- Assess daily weight, I/O, and signs of edema.
- Monitor vital signs closely, specifically BP.
- Assess deep tendon reflexes.
- Assess lung sounds for signs of pulmonary edema.
- Assess for headache unrelieved by medication, level of consciousness, neurological status for magnesium toxicity, and visual changes.
- Assess FHR.

 ALERT!

The antidote for magnesium sulfate is calcium gluconate administered via IVP over 5 to 10 minutes. This should always be available for any patient on magnesium sulfate. Toxicity symptoms include visual changes, flushing, muscle paralysis, and loss of deep tendon reflexes.

 POP QUIZ 5.3

The nurse is strictly monitoring the patient's I/O and has advocated for the IV fluids rate order to not be administered at more than 125 mL/hr. What complication is the nurse trying to prevent?

 POP QUIZ 5.4

A nurse is educating a pregnant patient on the risks of gestational hypertension. What symptoms could be mentioned?

MATERNAL HYPOVOLEMIA AND HEMORRHAGE

- *Maternal hypovolemia* is a decrease in the amount of circulating maternal blood volume.
- *Maternal hemorrhage* is the excessive loss of maternal blood.
- Causes of maternal hypovolemia include:
  - Anemia
  - Hemorrhage
- Causes of maternal hemorrhage include:
  - Placental abruption (see Placenta section)
  - Placenta previa
  - Unrepaired laceration from delivery (PPH after delivery of fetus)
  - Uterine rupture (see Uterus section)
- Both hypovolemia and hemorrhage lead to reduced maternal cardiac output, affecting placental perfusion. This leads to decreased blood flow to the fetus and decreased fetal oxygenation.

Nursing Interventions

- If fetus is still in utero:
  - Call for help.
  - Monitor patient:
    - Maintain continuous monitoring of FHR tracing; may observe late or prolonged decelerations or sinusoidal pattern, as well as minimal or absent FHR variability.
    - Monitor maternal vital signs.
    - Monitor uterine activity. Placental abruption can cause massive hemorrhage and usually causes uterine tenderness and rigidity; may observe tachycardia and/or increased uterine contractions (one after another) and hypotension.
  - Reposition patient into left lateral position.
  - Administer IV fluid bolus.
  - Administer supplemental oxygen.
    - Administer 10 L/min via nonrebreather face mask.
    - Discontinue as soon as possible based on fetal status.
  - Measure blood loss. QBL measurement is the preferred method.
  - Notify provider and initiate OB rapid response team (if applicable or available).
  - Prepare for administration of blood products:
    - Obtain IV access. May need a second IV line for blood administration.
    - Collect CBC and send type and screen labs.
    - Activate massive transfusion protocol if needed.
  - Prepare for emergent delivery.
  - Call for help.
  - Administer IV fluid bolus.
  - Monitor maternal vital signs for tachycardia and hypotension.
  - Initiate OB rapid response team (if available).
    - Assess the fundus. Massage if the fundus is boggy.

(continued)

Nursing Interventions *(continued)*

- Prepare for administration of blood products:
  - Obtain IV access.
  - Prepare a second IV line for blood administration (if needed).
  - Draw a CBC and send type and screen labs.
  - Activate massive transfusion protocol if indicated by large blood loss.
- Prepare to administer medications postpartum (Table 5.2):
  - Methylergonovine maleate
  - Carboprost tromethamine
  - Misoprostol
  - Oxytocin
  - Tranexamic acid
- Weigh all pads and linens for accurate blood loss (1 mL = 1 g).

 ALERT!

A pregnant patient who is hemorrhaging needs immediate delivery and fluid volume replacement.

Table 5.2 Medications for Postpartum Hemorrhage

Indications	Mechanism of Action	Contraindications, Precautions, and Adverse Effects
Semisynthetic ergot alkaloid derivatives (methylergonovine maleate)		
• PPH	• Stimulate contraction of the uterus to prevent or stop hemorrhage	• Medication is contraindicated in patients with hypertension or in patients who are allergic.
		• Use caution in patients with sepsis.
		• Adverse effects include hypertension, headache, abdominal pain, nausea, and vomiting.
Prostaglandin F2-alpha analogue (carboprost tromethamine)		
• PPH	• Stimulates contraction of the uterus to prevent or stop hemorrhage	• Medication is contraindicated in patients with asthma; acute pelvic inflammatory disease; or active cardiac, pulmonary, renal, or hepatic disease, and in patients who are allergic.
		• Adverse effects include fever, vomiting, severe diarrhea, nausea, flushing, headaches, and cough.

Table 5.2 Medications for Postpartum Hemorrhage *(continued)*

Indications	Mechanism of Action	Contraindications, Precautions, and Adverse Effects
Prostaglandin E1 analog (misoprostol)		
• PPH	• Stimulates contraction of the uterus to prevent or stop hemorrhage	• Medication is contraindicated in patients who are allergic. • Adverse effects include diarrhea, stomach pain, nausea, upset stomach, gas, and vaginal bleeding.
Cyclic nonapeptide hormone (oxytocin)		
• PPH	• Stimulates contraction of the uterus to prevent or stop hemorrhage	• Medication is contraindicated in patients who are allergic. • Adverse effects include nausea, vomiting, and more painful contractions.

INFERIOR VENA CAVA COMPRESSION

- Compression of the maternal IVC, especially during active labor, contributes to decreased cardiac output and maternal hypotension due to decreased venous return and hypoperfusion.
- Compression of the IVC can be due to maternal supine positioning during late pregnancy. In supine position, the weight of the fetus and uterus can mechanically compress the IVC; this compression is referred to as *IVC syndrome.*
- A contributing factor of IVC syndrome is an enlarged uterus. Maternal symptoms include lightheadedness, nausea, dizziness, shortness of breath, hypotension, and tachycardia.
- EFM tracing may show late decelerations, variable decelerations, prolonged decelerations, minimal or absent variability, and fetal bradycardia.

Nursing Interventions

- Maintain continuous FHR tracing.
- Reposition patient to correct fetal decelerations. Left lateral position can relieve IVC compression, which will improve fetal oxygenation and FHR.
- Administer IV fluid bolus.

 COMPLICATIONS

If not corrected, IVC compression can lead to decreased BP, thereby leading to late decelerations in the fetus and ultimately fetal death.

 ALERT!

An FHR tracing that indicates inadequate fetal oxygenation is an urgent situation because it is unknown how long the fetus has not been receiving adequate oxygen. If FHR variability is absent, the patient must be evaluated by the provider urgently. Interventions to improve fetal oxygenation (IV fluid bolus, position change) should be implemented, and the fetus may need to be delivered by cesarean section.

(continued)

Nursing Interventions *(continued)*

- Administer supplemental oxygen:
  - Administer 10 L/min via nonrebreather face mask.
  - Discontinue as soon as possible based on fetal status.
- Encourage modification of pushing efforts:
  - Push with every other or every third contraction.
  - Push while lying on side.
  - Temporarily discontinue pushing (during second stage labor).
- Evaluate fetal response to interventions.

 POP QUIZ 5.5

What are the risks associated with a pregnant patient lying in the supine position during the later weeks of the third trimester of pregnancy?

MATERNAL SEIZURE

- A *seizure* is a sudden, uncontrolled electrical disturbance in the brain.
- Seizures can cause changes in behavior, movements, feelings, and levels of consciousness.
- Two types of seizures are commonly seen during pregnancy:
  - *Focal*: Abnormal activity in one area of brain
  - *Generalized*: Affects the entire brain
- Maternal seizures can be harmful to the fetus due to the resulting increase in BP, decreased oxygenation, and electrolyte changes. The increase in intrauterine pressure during a seizure may also decrease uteroplacental blood flow.
- Causes:
  - Bleeding in the brain
  - Brain tumor
  - Eclampsia: Possible seizure when preeclampsia has progressed or is not controlled (preeclampsia can cause hypertension, proteinuria, hyperreflexia, headache, visual disturbances, and epigastric pain, and can progress to eclampsia)
  - Epilepsy
  - Hypertension
  - Stroke

Nursing Interventions

- Administer magnesium sulfate for eclamptic seizure (Table 5.3).
- Administer medication to treat severe hypertension in patients with preeclampsia (see Table 5.1):
  - Hydralazine
  - Nifedipine

 COMPLICATIONS

If not corrected, IVC compression can lead to decreased BP, thereby leading to late decelerations in the fetus and ultimately fetal death..

(continued)

Table 5.3 Medications for Preterm Labor

Indications	Mechanism of Action	Contraindications, Precautions, and Adverse Effects
Anticonvulsant (magnesium sulfate)		
• Neuroprotection in preterm neonate	• Exact mechanism unknown, but thought to: • Protect against inflammatory and oxidative injury • Stabilize BP and normalize cerebral blood flow • Stabilize neuronal membranes and block excitatory neurotransmitters	• Medication is contraindicated in patients with myasthenia gravis. • Adverse effects include flushing, nausea, diaphoresis, loss of deep tendon reflexes, respiratory depression, and cardiac arrest.
Beta adrenergic receptor agonists (isoproterenol, ritodrine)		
• Preterm labor	• Inhibit uterine contractions	• Medication is contraindicated in patients with tachycardia-sensitive cardiac disease and poorly controlled diabetes mellitus. • Adverse effects include tachycardia, hypotension, tremors, palpitations, shortness of breath, and chest pain.
Calcium channel blockers (nifedipine)		
• Preterm labor	• Relax the muscles in the uterus	• Medication is contraindicated in patients with hypotension and cardiac lesions. • Adverse effects include flushing, dizziness, hypotension, and slower heart rate.
Corticosteroid (betamethasone)		
• Lung maturity	• Causes release of surfactant	• Medication can increase blood sugar.
NSAID (indomethacin)		
• Preterm labor	• Blocks the production of prostaglandin, which causes contractions	• Medication is contraindicated in patients with platelet or bleeding disorders. • Adverse effects include nausea, vomiting, and reflux.

Nursing Interventions *(continued)*

- Maintain continuous monitoring of FHR; may observe:
  - Late decelerations
  - Minimal or absent variability
- Keep patient safe:
  - Monitor vital signs for return to baseline.
  - Monitor neurological status until returned to baseline.
  - Use padded side rails.
  - Remain with patient.

UTERUS

UTERINE RUPTURE

- *Uterine rupture* is a spontaneous tear in the uterus.
- Uterine rupture can cause massive maternal hemorrhage and severe fetal distress.
  - Uterine arteries may bleed out of uterus into abdomen.
  - Fetus can move out of uterus into abdomen.
- Causes of uterine rupture include:
  - Excessive use of uterotonics
  - Overdistention of uterus
  - Multifetal pregnancy
  - Polyhydramnios:
    - ○ Amnioinfusion with no fluid return out of vagina
    - ○ Uterine contractions
    - ○ Labor after a classical cesarean section
  - External cephalic version
  - Trial of labor after cesarean

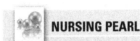

NURSING PEARL

Uteroplacental issues cause late decelerations.

Nursing Interventions

- Maintain continuous FHR tracing; may observe:
  - Bradycardia
  - Prolonged deceleration, late decelerations, or sinusoidal pattern
  - Minimal variability or absent variability
- Discontinue oxytocin, if applicable.
- Notify provider.
- Prepare for emergent cesarean section.

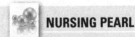

NURSING PEARL

Always maintain clear, closed-loop communication with the OB team and providers when providing maternal stabilization.

- Prepare for PPH after delivery.
- Prepare to administer postpartum medications (see Table 5.2):
  - Methylergonovine maleate
  - Carboprost tromethamine
  - Misoprostol
  - Oxytocin
  - Tranexamic acid

 ALERT!

If a patient is pushing and the head is at +3 station and then suddenly goes back to -1 station, call provider immediately due to symptoms of uterine rupture.

EXCESSIVE UTERINE ACTIVITY (TACHYSYSTOLE)

- *Excessive uterine activity*, also known as *tachysystole*, is defined as more than five contractions in 10 minutes.
- Excessive uterine activity causes *increased uterine resting tone*, which is pressure within the uterus when it is not contracting. This can impair placental circulation and lead to decreased FHR variability.
- When excessive uterine activity occurs, the FHR may show minimal, late, variable, or prolonged decelerations.
  - Figure 5.1 shows an FHR tracing demonstrating variable decelerations with absent to minimal variability.
  - Note the frequency of the uterine contractions.
- Causes of excessive uterine activity are unknown, but may include:
  - Cervical ripening agents
  - Chorioamnionitis
  - Maternal dehydration
  - Oxytocin
  - Placental abruption
  - Uterine rupture

Nursing Interventions

- Maintain continuous monitoring of FHR tracing; may observe late, variable, or prolonged decelerations.
- Decrease or discontinue oxytocin if it is being administered.
- Administer supplemental oxygen:
  - Administer 10 L/min via nonrebreather face mask.
  - Discontinue as soon as possible based on fetal status.
- Administer tocolytics per order, with the following objectives:
  - Return uterine activity to normal spacing of contractions.
  - Decrease the uterine resting tone to the normal range.
- Administer IV fluid bolus or increase IV fluid rate per order.

 POP QUIZ 5.6

A 34-year-old patient gave birth to their fifth baby 2 hours ago and has not been able to void since delivery. The patient calls for help because they passed a large egg-sized clot and are still leaking blood. An assessment finds a boggy fundus, but it is located +2 and to the right. What is the likely cause and the appropriate intervention?

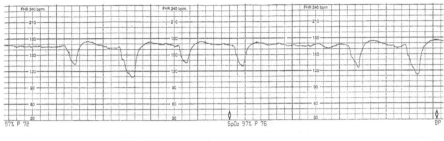

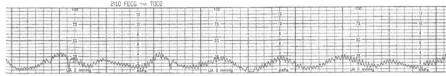

Figure 5.1 Excessive uterine activity with variable decelerations.

Source: Murray, M., Huelsmann, G., & Koperski, N. (2019). *Essentials of fetal and uterine monitoring.* Springer Publishing Company.

PLACENTA

ABRUPTIO PLACENTA

- *Abruptio placenta* is the complete or partial separation of the placenta from the uterine wall. This can happen in two ways:
  - Partial (chronic): May be able to stabilize without complications
  - Complete: Requires emergent delivery
- Abruptio placenta compromises fetal oxygenation due to collapse or destruction of the intervillous space and interference with the fetal supply of oxygen and nutrients.

 ALERT!

Diabetes affects the development of and the function of the placenta. Nurses should be aware that maternal blood sugar may need to be assessed.

- Abruptio placenta can be reflected on FHR tracing by a sinusoidal fetal heart pattern, which reflects fetal compromise from decreased oxygenation (Figure 5.2).
- Causes of abruption include:
  - Abdominal trauma
  - Cocaine use
  - High BP
  - Preeclampsia and eclampsia
- Symptoms include:
  - Heavy vaginal bleeding
  - Hypotension
  - Maternal tachycardia
  - Severe abdominal pain
  - Rigid abdomen

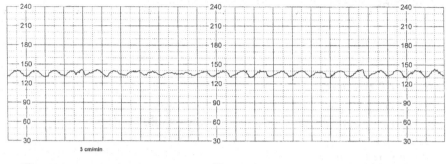

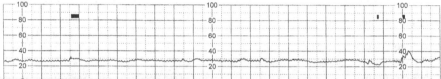

Figure 5.2 This FHR tracing is from a 29-year-old patient being evaluated after a motor vehicle crash. The patient's abdomen is hard and painful, and the patient is experiencing vaginal bleeding. This tracing is a sinusoidal pattern, likely due to a placental abruption caused by the motor vehicle crash.

Source: Murray, M., Huelsmann, G., & Koperski, N. (2019). *Essentials of fetal and uterine monitoring.* Springer Publishing Company.

Nursing Interventions

- Call for help.
- Monitor blood loss; if patient is visibly bleeding, measure pads and linens for accurate blood loss (1 mL = 1 g).
- Monitor vital signs for signs of shock, including tachycardia and hypotension.
- Maintain continuous FHR tracing; may observe late or prolonged decelerations or sinusoidal pattern, bradycardia, or minimal or absent FHR variability.
- Reposition patient to left lateral position.
- Obtain IV access and administer IV fluid bolus.
- Administer supplemental oxygen:
  - Administer 10 L/min via nonrebreather face mask.
  - Discontinue as soon as possible based on fetal status.
- Collect blood for CBC and type and screen labs.
- Prepare for possible emergent delivery.

PLACENTAL IMPLANTATION COMPLICATIONS

- Placenta accreta is a serious complication.
- The placenta implants too deeply into the uterus and:

(continued)

PLACENTAL IMPLANTATION COMPLICATIONS *(continued)*

- Can invade the muscles of the uterus (placenta increta).
- Can grow through the uterine wall (placenta percreta).
- Will require cesarean section to deliver fetus and possible hysterectomy.

Causes and Risk Factors

- Advanced maternal age
- Previous childbirth (increased risk with each delivery)
- Previous uterine surgery

Nursing Interventions

- Prepare for blood transfusion.
- Prepare for cesarean section and possible hysterectomy.
- Provide emotional support.

POP QUIZ 5.7

A 19-year-old patient presents to labor and delivery (L&D) in excruciating abdominal pain with a large amount of bright-red vaginal bleeding and appears to be pregnant and close to full term. The patient has not had prenatal care. What is an appropriate assessment, and what nursing interventions are needed?

UMBILICAL CORD

NUCHAL CORD

- Nuchal cord occurs when the umbilical cord wraps around the fetus's neck while in utero.
- The umbilical cord may be loosely or tightly wrapped around the fetus's neck one or more times.
- Complications are more likely to occur if the nuchal cord is tight.
- Nuchal cord can be an incidental finding at birth.
- Nuchal cord can cause recurrent variable decelerations.

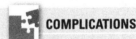

COMPLICATIONS

Up to 20% of fetal demise autopsies demonstrate fatal compromise of umbilical cord circulation.

Causes

- Fetal size or movements:
  - Small preterm fetus
  - Fetus that flipped from breech to vertex
- Possible differential flow patterns in umbilical cord

Nursing Interventions

- Monitor fetus using continuous EFM.
- Perform interventions related to fetal heart tracing, if indicated (Figure 5.3).
  - Change patient position.
  - Administer IV fluid bolus.
  - Administer oxygen.
  - Notify provider.
  - Prepare for cesarean section delivery, if required.

ALERT!

Cord compression and umbilical cord prolapse can also cause variable decelerations.

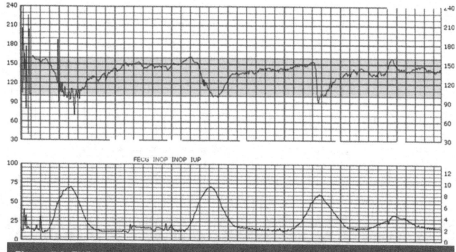

Figure 5.3 FHR showing a possible nuchal cord. This is a category II FHR with a baseline of 150 bpm, moderate variability, no accelerations, and variable decelerations.

Source: Nye, R. (2019). *Essentials of fetal heart rate monitoring.* Springer Publishing Company. https://doi.org/10.189 1/9780826174246.0006

UMBILICAL CORD COMPRESSION

- *Umbilical cord compression* is mechanical pressure on the umbilical cord from the fetus.
- Umbilical cord compression induces fetal baroceptor stimulation and parasympathetic response, causing variable decelerations in the FHR, as well as minimal or absent variability.
- Umbilical cord compression can be caused by:
  - Cord wrapped around fetal body
  - Cord wrapped around fetal neck
  - Fetus holding onto the cord
  - Oligohydramnios
  - Position of fetus
- Umbilical cord compression causes a transient disruption of the maternal–fetal oxygen pathway and can block blood flow.

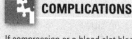 **COMPLICATIONS**

If compression or a blood clot blocks the UV, the fetus could suffer permanent injury or even death.

Nursing Interventions

- Maintain continuous FHR tracing; may observe variable decelerations (Figure 5.4).
- Reposition patient to correct variable decelerations and relieve cord compression:
  - Hands and knees position
  - Left or right lateral position

(continued)

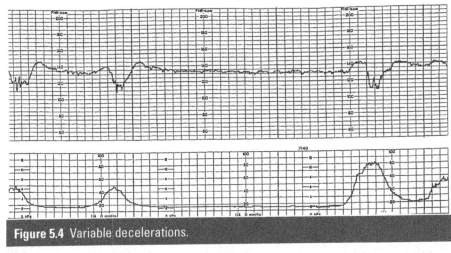

Figure 5.4 Variable decelerations.

Source: Murray, M., Huelsmann, G., & Koperski, N. (2019). *Essentials of fetal and uterine monitoring.* Springer Publishing Company.

Nursing Interventions *(continued)*

- Administer IV fluid bolus.
- Administer supplemental oxygen:
  - Administer 10 L/min via nonrebreather face mask.
  - Discontinue as soon as possible based on fetal status.
- Encourage modification of pushing efforts during labor:
  - Pushing with every other or every third contraction
  - Pushing on side
  - Temporary discontinuation of pushing
- Evaluate fetal response to interventions.
- Prepare for amnioinfusion:
  - *Amnioinfusion* is a treatment for persistent variable decelerations in the presence of ruptured membranes.
  - Amnioinfusion is used to increase fluid volume via the infusion of normal sterile saline through the cervix.
  - Observe for fluid return from the vagina on the underpad. Fluid that is administered must be discharged from the vagina. If there is no fluid return, turn off amnioinfusion to prevent uterine rupture.

UMBILICAL CORD PROLAPSE

- *Umbilical cord prolapse* occurs when the umbilical cord enters the birth canal through the cervix ahead of the fetus.
- A prolapsed cord can cause obstruction of blood flow through the umbilical cord, which can affect fetal oxygenation and fetal blood flow.

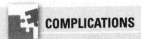 **COMPLICATIONS**

Umbilical cord prolapse causes mechanical cord compression due to pressure from the fetus and stretching of the cord, leading to compromised fetal oxygen supply.

- A sign of umbilical cord prolapse is when the cord can be seen or palpated on examination.
- FHR tracing may show:
  - Fetal bradycardia
  - Variable or prolonged decelerations
- Causes of umbilical cord prolapse include:
  - Rupture of membranes before 32 weeks' gestation
  - Premature, artificial, or spontaneous rupture of membranes
  - Greater or equal to 4 cm cervical dilation
  - Higher fetal station: Fetal head not well engaged in the pelvic inlet
  - Malpresentation of fetus (e.g., breech or transverse position)

Nursing Interventions

- Maintain continuous monitoring of FHR tracing.
- Assess for pulsating umbilical cord presence in vagina.
- Reposition and elevate fetus off the cord manually.
- Reposition patient in Trendelenburg position.
- Notify provider and prepare for emergent operative delivery (cesarean section).

 ALERT!

During an umbilical cord prolapse, the nurse may observe variable or prolonged decelerations or fetal bradycardia.

FETUS

HYPOXIA/ACIDOSIS

- Hypoxia occurs prior to labor or during labor and delivery when:
  - Fetal oxygen is impaired.
  - A persistent category II FHR tracing, lasting longer than 60 minutes with minimal or absent variability, indicates possible hypoxia.
  - A category I tracing changes to category III, which is indicative of an acute hypoxic event (Figure 5.5).
- Acidosis occurs with excessive buildup of hydrogen in tissues.
  - Acidosis is caused by fetal hypoxia.
  - Acidosis can cause long-term morbidity.

Causes and Risk Factors

- Maternal cigarette smoking
- Fetal anemia
- Maternal cardiovascular disease
- Maternal respiratory condition
- Placental abruption

(continued)

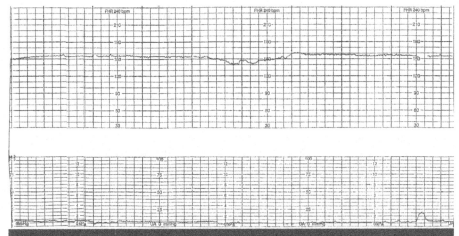

Figure 5.5. FHR with absent variability, a spontaneous deceleration, and no accelerations demonstrates fetal hypoxia. This is a category III FHR that needs immediate interventions. The nurse should call the provider, get help to start an IV and give IV fluid bolus, reposition the patient, and administer oxygen.

Source: Murray, M., Huelsmann, G., & Koperski, N. (2019). *Essentials of fetal and uterine monitoring.* Springer Publishing Company, LLC.

Causes and Risk Factors *(continued)*

- Placental infarction
- Preeclampsia
- Prolapsed or occluded umbilical cord

Nursing Interventions

- Monitor fetus using continuous EFM.
- Perform interventions if category II or III FHR tracing:
  - Change patient position.
  - Administer IV fluid bolus.
  - Administer oxygen 8 to 10 L per mask.
  - Notify provider.
  - Prepare for cesarean section delivery, if required.
- Obtain a cord blood gas sample from the umbilical cord:
  - Collect from UA first, then UV.
  - Difference in artery and vein gases may give further information on duration:

 ALERT!

Cord blood gases (UA and UV) can help to determine whether the hypoxia is occurring before or during labor.

○ In placental dysfunction where hypoxia is due to reduced placental transfer, UA and UV values will both be abnormal and similar.
○ In acute cord compression or fetal bradycardia, hypoxia and acidosis will be predominantly in the UA, leading to a large arteriovenous difference. This difference can help to determine when acidosis occurred.
● Results show fetal oxygenation status at time of delivery.
● Results can help the neonatal care team to understand the effectiveness of organ function and the ability of the baby to compensate for acute or chronic changes at the moment of birth.

SHOULDER DYSTOCIA

● *Shoulder dystocia* occurs when one or both fetal shoulders is impacted behind the symphysis pubis, or when descent of the fetal shoulder is obstructed by the sacral promontory after delivery of head.
● Shoulder dystocia results in prolonged delivery; the time from delivery of head to delivery of body is more than 60 seconds.

 COMPLICATIONS

In the neonate, brachial plexus injury and clavicle and humerus fractures are possible. Hypoxic ischemic brain injury or death can occur. In the patient, vaginal lacerations, uterine rupture, or PPH can occur.

Causes and Risk Factors

● May be indeterminate
● Larger than average fetus (greater than 4,000 g)
● Maternal risk factors:
  ● Abnormal pelvic anatomy
  ● Advanced age
  ● Diabetes
  ● Macrosomic fetus
  ● Multiparity
  ● Obesity and excessive gestational weight gain
  ● Postterm pregnancy
  ● Previous shoulder dystocia
  ● Short stature

 ALERT!

A prolonged second stage of labor may be predictive of a shoulder dystocia and should alert the nurse to have extra help available.

Nursing Interventions

● Prepare to have extra nurses present at delivery if a large fetus (greater than 4,000 g) is expected based on ultrasound or Leopold's maneuver.
● Prepare for delivery with resuscitation equipment and appropriate personnel for neonate.
● Stay calm.

 ALERT!

The turtle sign (fetal head, usually dark red or purple, appearing and retracting during pushing) suggests a possible shoulder dystocia.

(continued)

Nursing Interventions *(continued)*

- Assist provider with maneuvers:
  - Primary maneuvers:
    - McRoberts (performed by nurse with provider):
      - Rotation of the pelvis helps free the impacted shoulder.
      - Remove pillows and lower head of bed so patient is flat in the supine position.
      - Hyperflex patient's legs against abdomen and bring knees toward patient's ears.
    - Suprapubic pressure:
      - Abduction and rotation of the anterior shoulder decreases diameter of fetal shoulders going under the symphysis pubis.
      - Firm and steady downward and lateral pressure is applied above the pubic bone with the palm or fist to the posterior aspect of the anterior shoulder.
      - Application of pressure is easier when standing on stool above patient.
  - Secondary maneuvers; all except Gaskin maneuver are performed by provider:
    - Gaskin maneuver: Patient is placed on hands and knees to increase diameter of pelvis.
    - Posterior axilla sling traction: Double-looped sling using a suction catheter or urinary catheter is inserted under the posterior fetal axilla, and traction is used to deliver the shoulder.
    - Rubin maneuver: Provider pushes behind most accessible shoulder toward fetus's chest, reducing diameter of shoulders.
    - Woods screw maneuver: Posterior shoulder is rotated to free anterior shoulder.
  - Desperation maneuvers: Performed by provider as last attempt, due to increased maternal and fetal morbidity and mortality:
    - Intentional breaking of fetal clavicle
    - Zavanelli maneuver: Replacing the fetal head in the vagina and performing cesarean section
- Ensure that all maneuvers performed are included in delivery documentation.

NURSING PEARL

The key to managing complications is to be prepared. Practice for emergencies by performing simulation drills. When complications occur, remain calm and get help.

POP QUIZ 5.8

A 37-year-old patient with gestational diabetes is in L&D for induction of labor due to uncontrolled blood sugars. Height is 4'10, and weight is 220 lb. The abdomen appears large. The patient is 10 cm dilated and starts pushing. What should the nurse caring for this patient do?

OTHER MATERNAL COMPLICATIONS

CHORIOAMNIONITIS

- *Chorioamnionitis* is an infection of the amniotic sac, most often bacterial in origin.
- Chorioamnionitis occurs in about 4% of deliveries at term but occurs more frequently in preterm deliveries and with premature rupture of membranes.
- A major risk factor for chorioamnionitis is prolonged rupture of membranes.
- Signs and symptoms include:
  - Fetal tachycardia
  - Foul-smelling amniotic fluid
  - Maternal fever
  - Uterine tenderness
- Chorioamnionitis is a risk factor for both maternal and neonatal sequelae.
  - Neonatal complications include:
    - ○ Bronchopulmonary dysplasia in premature infants
    - ○ Cerebral palsy
    - ○ Neonatal death
    - ○ Neonatal sepsis
    - ○ Neurologic abnormalities
    - ○ Premature birth
    - ○ Respiratory distress syndrome
    - ○ Retinopathy of prematurity
  - Maternal complications include:
    - ○ Maternal sepsis
    - ○ Operative delivery
    - ○ PPH
    - ○ Preterm delivery
    - ○ Severe pelvic infections
    - ○ Subcutaneous wound infections

Causes

- Existing infection such as:
  - *Candida*
  - *Escherichia coli*
  - Group B *Streptococcus*
  - Trichomoniasis
- Multiple vaginal examinations after rupture of membranes
- Prolonged rupture of membranes

Nursing Interventions

- Administer antibiotics and antipyretics as ordered.
- Monitor maternal temperature frequently, per institutional policy.
- Use continuous fetal monitoring to assess for FHR complications.
- Send placenta cultures to lab after delivery, as ordered by provider.

POSTPARTUM HEMORRHAGE

- PPH is characterized as a cumulative blood loss of 1,000 mL or more after delivery.
- Measuring blood loss is a key component of recognizing PPH; estimation is inaccurate.
- PPH may occur immediately after birth or up to 12 weeks after delivery.
- PPH needs immediate intervention and treatment.
- Medications used for PPH (see Table 5.2):
  - Carboprost tromethamine
  - Methylergonovine maleate
  - Misoprostol
  - Oxytocin
  - Tranexamic acid
- Other treatments include:
  - Blood replacement
    - RBCs
    - FFP
    - Platelets
  - Emptying of bladder
  - Fundal massage
  - IV fluid replacement
  - Removal of retained placenta
  - Repair of lacerations
  - Surgical interventions:
    - Hysterectomy
    - Uterine artery embolization
    - Uterine compression sutures

 NURSING PEARL

Use a "bundle" that helps to recognize and treat PPH. Evidence-based patient safety bundles provide algorithms and instructions for caring for a patient who is hemorrhaging.

 COMPLICATIONS

PPH can be life threatening and needs immediate attention.

 COMPLICATIONS

PPH is the leading cause of maternal mortality in the world. Early recognition is imperative.

Causes and Risk Factors

- Atony of the uterus
  - Causes and risk factors:
    - Distended (full) bladder
    - Infection
    - Large fetus
    - Medication (use of magnesium sulfate or prolonged use of oxytocin)
    - Multiparous patient
    - Multiple gestation
- Bleeding or clotting disorder; may not be diagnosed prior to giving birth
- Retained tissue
  - Placental fragments or amniotic membrane remain in uterus.
  - Small placental fragments can lead to delayed PPH.

- Trauma
  - Hematoma: Collection of blood can occur from forceps or vacuum use.
  - Lacerations of the vagina or cervix that are not completely repaired can continue to bleed, leading to hemorrhage.

Nursing Interventions

- Administer medications as ordered.
- Administer oxygen if needed.
- Apply Foley or straight catheter if needed.
- Assist with tamponade insertion if used.
- Request assistance from additional nurses and provider and assign roles.
- Measure QBL:
  - Weigh pads and linens.
  - Subtract dry weight from blood-soaked weight to calculate QBL.
  - 1g = 1 mL blood.
- Perform fundal checks for uterine tone after delivery per protocol.
- When observing blood loss, always roll the patient and check for pooled blood under the buttocks.
- Perform fundal massage.
- Prepare patient for operating room as necessary.
- Provide an IV fluid bolus.
- Remain with the patient.

 NURSING PEARL

During fundal checks, the fundus should continue to contract and be felt at the same location or lower. If the fundal height increases or is palpated to the left or right (instead of midline), a full bladder should be suspected. The patient should void or may require catheterization.

DIABETES MELLITUS

- Two types of diabetes mellitus can be seen during pregnancy:
  - GDM
    - *GDM* refers to carbohydrate intolerance that develops during pregnancy.
    - A patient whose GDM is controlled by diet can be further classified as A1GDM, whereas a patient who requires medication can be classified as A2GDM.
  - Pregestational diabetes mellitus:
    - Refers to a patient who is already diagnosed with diabetes before becoming pregnant
    - Affects 1% to 2% of all pregnant patients
    - Type 1:
      - Thought to be an autoimmune reaction that destroys the cells in the pancreas that make insulin
      - Requires insulin administration
    - Type 2:
      - Cells do not respond to insulin properly.
      - The pancreas produces more insulin in an attempt to fulfill cell requirements.
      - The pancreas is unable to keep up insulin production, and blood sugar rises.
- Diabetes can cause increased risk of spontaneous abortion, congenital defects, and stillbirth. Increased fetal surveillance is necessary.

Causes and Risk Factors

- Pregestational:
  - Type 1: Family history
  - Type 2:
    - Age older than 45 years
    - Family history
    - GDM during previous pregnancy
    - African American, Hispanic/Latinx, American Indian, or Alaska Native descent
    - Obesity
    - Physically active less than three times per week
- Gestational:
  - Age older than 25 years
  - Family history of type 2 diabetes mellitus
  - African American, Hispanic/Latinx, American Indian, Alaska Native, Native Hawaiian, or Pacific Islander descent
  - GDM during previous pregnancy
  - Has given birth to baby over 9 lbs
  - History of polycystic ovary syndrome
  - Obesity

Nursing Interventions

- Monitor maternal blood sugars per hospital policy.
- Monitor fetal status per hospital policy.

OBESITY

- Obesity is characterized by a BMI that is 30 or higher.
- Maternal obesity may be associated with certain conditions in the fetus:
  - Birth defects
  - Childhood asthma
  - Childhood obesity
  - Macrosomia
- Maternal complications of obesity may include GDM, hypertension (and preeclampsia), miscarriage, sleep apnea, and cesarean section with risk of cesarean section complications, such as wound infections.

Causes

- Genetics
- Thyroid disease
- Dietary habits

Nursing Interventions

- Educate patient about weight gain early in pregnancy.
- No interventions are provided in L&D.

COMPLICATIONS OF LABOR

For normal uterine activity, see the end of Chapter 4.

FAILURE TO PROGRESS

- *Failure to progress* is defined as:
  - Active labor (greater than or equal to 6 cm dilated) after rupture of membranes, but with no cervical change after 4 hours of adequate uterine contractions
  - Rupture of membranes but no cervical change after 6 hours of inadequate contractions with use of oxytocin
- *Prolonged latent phase of labor* (less than 6 cm dilated) is defined as more than 20 hours for a primiparous patient or more than 14 hours for a multiparous patient.
- *Arrest of labor in second stage* is defined as multiparous patient pushing for at least 2 hours or primiparous patient pushing for at least 3 hours.

Causes

- Excessive maternal weight gain
- Induction of labor
- Macrosomic fetus
- Malpresentation of fetus
- Psychological issues (stress, anxiety, fear)
- Small maternal pelvis

Nursing Interventions

- Assist provider with manual fetal rotation.
- Assist provider with operative vaginal delivery.
- Provide continuous labor support.

OPERATIVE DELIVERY

- *Cesarean section* is operative delivery through surgical incision in the patient's abdomen. There is an increased risk of maternal morbidity due to possible:
  - Hemorrhage
  - Infection
  - Placental complications with future pregnancies
- *Operative vaginal delivery* is delivery with use of forceps or vacuum.
  - Lower risk of maternal complications than with cesarean section
  - Complications for neonate not greater than those with cesarean section

Causes

- Failure to progress
- Macrosomic infant
- Malpresentation of fetus
- Maternal infection

(continued)

Causes *(continued)*

- Multiple gestation
- Nonreassuring FHR

Nursing Interventions

- Assist provider as needed.
- Prepare patient for operative vaginal delivery. Instruct patient to listen to provider and push when directed.
- Prepare patient for cesarean section:
  - Abdominal prep: Remove hair with hair clippers.
  - Clean skin according to institutional protocol.
  - Provide emotional support.
  - Obtain IV access.
  - Move patient to operating room when ready.

PRETERM LABOR

- *Preterm labor* is defined as birth between 20 0/7 weeks of gestation and 36 6/7 weeks of gestation.
- It is the leading cause of neonatal mortality and the most common reason for antenatal hospitalization.

Causes and Risk Factors

- Age younger than 17 or older than 35 years
- Alcohol use
- Cigarette smoking
- Diabetes
- Drug use
- History of preterm birth
- Hypertensive disorders
- Infection
  - Amniotic fluid
  - Lower genital tract
- Interval of less than 6 months between pregnancies
- In vitro fertilization
- Multiple gestation
- Stressful events
- Trauma
- Uterus, cervix, or placenta problems

Nursing Interventions

- Administer medication as ordered.
- Treatment includes:
  - Single course of corticosteroids recommended for pregnant patients between 24 and 34 weeks of gestation who are at risk of delivery within 7 days

- First-line tocolytic treatment with beta-adrenergic receptor agonists, calcium channel blockers, or NSAIDs for short-term prolongation of pregnancy (see Table 5.3)
- Tocolytic therapy to possibly prolong pregnancy long enough to administer antenatal corticosteroids and magnesium sulfate for neuroprotection
- Educate patient on recognizing signs of preterm labor.
- Monitor FHR and contractions.

RESOURCES

American College of Obstetricians and Gynecologists. (2016a). Obstetric care consensus: Safe prevention of the primary cesarean delivery. *Obstetrics & Gynecology, 123*(3), 693–711. https://doi .org/10.1097/01.aog.0000444441.04111.1d

American College of Obstetricians and Gynecologists. (2016b). Practice bulletin No. 171: Management of preterm labor. *Obstetrics & Gynecology, 128*(4), pe155–pe164. https://doi.org/10.1 097/aog.0000000000001711

American College of Obstetricians and Gynecologists. (2017). Practice bulletin No. 183: Postpartum hemorrhage. *Obstetrics & Gynecology, 130*(4), pe168–pe186. https://doi.org/10.1097/aog.0000000 000002351

American College of Obstetricians and Gynecologists. (2018a). American College of Obstetricians and Gynecologists practice bulletin no. 190: Gestational diabetes mellitus. *Obstetrics & Gynecology, 131*(2), pe49–pe64. https://doi.org/10.1097/aog.0000000000002501

American College of Obstetricians and Gynecologists. (2018b). American College of Obstetricians and Gynecologists practice bulletin No. 201 summary: Pregestational diabetes mellitus. *Obstetrics & Gynecology, 132*(6), 1514–1516. https://doi.org/10.1097/aog.0000000000002961

American College of Obstetricians and Gynecologists. (2019). Executive summary. *Obstetrics & Gynecology, 123*(4), 896–901. https://doi.org/10.1097/01.aog.0000445580.65983.d2

American College of Obstetricians and Gynecologists. (2020). Gestational hypertension and preeclampsia. *Obstetrics & Gynecology, 135*(6), pe237–pe260. https://doi.org/10.1097/aog.000000 0000003891

Conde-Agudelo, A., Romero, R., Jung, E. J., & Sánchez, Garcia, Á, J. (2020). Management of clinical chorioamnionitis: An evidence-based approach. *American Journal of Obstetrics and Gynecology, 223*(6), 848–869. https://doi.org/10.1016/j.ajog.2020.09.044

Holland, T. (2020). Shoulder dystocia. *Nursing Made Incredibly Easy! 18*(6), 9–14. https://doi.org/ 10.1097/01.nme.0000717680.73079.f8

Mayo Foundation for Medical Education and Research. (2020a). *Placenta accreta.* https://www.mayocl inic.org/diseases-conditions/placenta-accreta/symptoms-causes/syc-20376431

Mayo Foundation for Medical Education and Research. (2020b). *Placental abruption.* https://www. mayoclinic.org/diseases-conditions/placental-abruption/symptoms-causes/syc-20376458

Moldenhauer, J. S. (2020). *Uterine rupture—Gynecology and obstetrics.* Merck Manuals Professional Edition. https://www.merckmanuals.com/professional/gynecology-and-obstetrics/ abnormalities-and-complications-of-labor-and-delivery/uterine-rupture#:~:text=Uterine%20rupt ure%20is%20spontaneous%20tearing%20of%20the%20uterus,in%20women%20who%20have%20 had%20prior%20cesarean%20deliveries

Murray, M., Huelsmann, G., & Koperski, N. (2019). *Essentials of fetal and uterine monitoring* (sec. 4). Springer Publishing Company.

National Institute for Health and Care Excellence. (2019). *Hypertension in pregnancy: Diagnosis and management.* https://www.nice.org.uk/guidance/ng133

Nye, R. (2019). *Essentials of fetal heart rate monitoring.* Springer Publishing Company. https://doi.org/ 10.1891/9780826174246.0006

Peesay, M. (2017). Nuchal cord and its implications. *Maternal Health, Neonatology and Perinatology*, *3*(1), 28. https://doi.org/10.1186/s40748-017-0068-7

Prescribers' Digital Reference. (n.d.). *Invanz [Drug Information]*. https://www.pdr.net/drug-information/invanz?druglabelid=359

Sayed Ahmed, W. A., & Hamdy, M. A. (2018). Optimal management of umbilical cord prolapse. *International Journal of Women's Health, 10*, 459–465. https://doi.org/10.2147/IJWH.S130879

6

PROFESSIONAL ISSUES

OVERVIEW

Ethical and legal issues, along with patient safety and QI, have important implications in obstetric nursing. This chapter covers these key points:

- Ethical decision-making plays a role in the care of the pregnant patient and fetus.
- Legal implications affect the care of the patient and fetus. Obstetrics is a high-risk, high-liability area of nursing and medicine.
- The safety of the patient and fetus must always be considered a priority.
- QI is an ongoing process to improve care for the patient.

ETHICS

Overview

- Four principles are used to address ethical issues, problems, and dilemmas: beneficence, justice, nonmaleficence, and respect for patient autonomy.
- *Beneficence* is doing good and providing care that benefits the patient. *Example:* The nurse who is caring for a patient in labor provides a massage to help with pain management.
- *Justice* is the principle of rendering to others what is due to them. *Example:* The medical staff uses a triage system to determine which patient receives care first.
- *Nonmaleficence* is an obligation to not cause harm or injury. *Example:* If a nurse is working while impaired, it is the responsibility of any nurse working with the impaired nurse to report them.
- *Respect for patient autonomy* acknowledges an individual's right to hold views, to make choices, and to act based on their own personal values and beliefs.
  - Respect for autonomy provides a foundation for informed consent. Informed consent requires that staff adequately inform patients about their medical condition and the available therapies. Informed consent must be obtained by the provider with a witness present during the time of the consent and the patient signature.
    - ○ The provider needs to ensure that the patient understands all risks, benefits, and consequences in order to make an informed decision.
    - ○ The patient then chooses whether or not to receive the specific treatment(s).

(continued)

Overview *(continued)*

- Respect for patient autonomy must consider the pregnant patient and the fetus (or fetuses), which may present conflicts between or among ethical principles. Examples include:
  - A pregnant patient may initially refuse to have an induction of labor. However, if the patient goes past 42 weeks' gestation, the recommendation for an induction will come from the provider because of the potential danger to the fetus in both postterm gestation and delivery. Although the patient has refused the induction, they may ultimately agree when they understand the potential risks to the fetus. The patient may feel as if they do not have a choice. In this example, the ethical principal of patient autonomy is in conflict with the ethical principle of nonmaleficence.
  - A patient in labor initially refuses a cesarean section. However, the fetal heart tracing reveals fetal bradycardia that does not improve with interventions. In this case, the provider states that the fetus will need to be delivered by an emergent cesarean section, which places the ethical principal of patient autonomy in conflict with the ethical principle of nonmaleficence.

Nursing Interventions

- Advocate for the patient.
- Contact hospital chaplain/clergy for spiritual care, as appropriate.
- Escalate to the ethics committee as needed.
- Follow the institution's policies and procedures.
- Provide emotional support to the patient and family members.
- Recognize signs and symptoms of moral distress.
- Report unethical and unsafe situations.
- Use the chain of command in situations when caring for a patient causes an ethical issue.
- Participate in code/event debrief to share experiences and identify opportunities for improvement.
- Review organizational guidelines for situations involving the nurse's personal or professional values (conscientious objection) in the care of maternal and neonatal complications.

 POP QUIZ 6.1

A nurse is caring for a patient who has developed a birth plan that includes delayed bathing of the neonate. The nurse tells the patient that they cannot follow the birth plan because they need to bathe the newborn right away. What ethical principle applies to this situation?

 POP QUIZ 6.2

An nurse volunteers at a clinic for underserved patients. What ethical principle is the nurse following?

LEGALITY

Overview

- Obstetrics is a high-litigation specialty.
- Complications leading to injury or death of a pregnant patient and/or a fetus may lead to legal action.
- Families have 1 to 12 years after birth to initiate legal action, depending on the state they live in.
- Nurses may be named in lawsuits.
- Nurses must remain competent in their field. *Nursing competence* is the ability to safely perform functions that demonstrate essential knowledge and skills that comply with the standard of care.
- Critical nursing skills include:
  - Analyzing and interpreting FHR tracings and uterine contraction patterns
  - Acting in response to the physiology of fetal heart patterns and responding to/intervening in issues causing abnormal FHR tracings and uterine contraction patterns
  - Acting to prevent injury to the patient and the fetus
  - Advocating for and promoting the safety of the patient and the fetus
  - Appropriately implementing and updating the plan of care and ensuring that the patient understands the plan of care
  - Determining a nursing diagnosis and implementing a plan of care and interventions based on the nursing diagnosis
  - Determining the physiologic meaning and implications of the FHR and uterine contraction patterns
  - Identifying and treating potential risks to the patient and the fetus
- *Standard of care* is defined as the behavior of an ordinary, careful, reasonable, or prudent nurse.
  - Some examples include:
    - Anticipating potential problems with the patient and/or fetus
    - Collaborating with other members of the healthcare team to ensure safe patient care of the patient and/or fetus
    - Developing a comprehensive plan of care supported by evidence-based practice
    - Evaluating and reevaluating effectiveness of care
    - Evaluating the need for immediate intervention and responding appropriately
    - Identifying problems and developing interventions based on correct interpretation of the data
    - Implementing a plan of care efficiently and safely
  - Investigating reasons for abnormal FHR patterns by obtaining all necessary data and implementing appropriate and timely interventions
  - An important standard of care is the competent and safe analysis of FHR patterns and uterine contraction patterns.
  - *Substandard intrapartal care* is defined as a provider failing to give care that meets the appropriate standards of care.

(continued)

Overview *(continued)*

- ○ Not responding to or failing to respond in a timely manner to an FHR tracing showing signs of distress may be associated with fetal complications.
- ○ Failing to intervene when a fetus has signs of oxygen deprivation, such as absent variability and repetitive late decelerations, is considered substandard care.
- ○ A lawsuit related to substandard care may assess whether the nurse:
    - ▪ Identified and documented an abnormal FHR tracing
    - ▪ Responded appropriately to the FHR tracing, according to guidelines
    - ▪ Communicated the appropriate information to the provider in a timely manner
    - • Used the chain of command
- Sources of information that contribute to the determination of the standard of care include:
    - ○ Collaborative agreements
    - ○ Hospital bylaws, rules, and regulations
    - ○ Institutional policies, procedures, and protocols
    - ○ Publications, such as textbooks, journals, committee opinions, and practice bulletins; state licensure practice acts or rules and regulations
    - ○ Professional organizations that create guidelines in the obstetrics and neonatal settings (AWHONN, ACOG, and AORN)
- Nurses must advocate for those who are not able to advocate for themselves due to fear, lack of knowledge, or inability.
- *Negligence* includes the concepts of duty, breach of duty, causation, and damages.
    - • *Duty* is to optimize outcomes and prevent injury.
    - • *Breach of duty* is the failure to meet the standard of care, which prevents fulfillment of the duty to prevent injury.
    - • *Causation* is the direct connection between the failure to meet the standard of care and the injury.
    - • *Damages* can result in monetary compensation for the patient.
        - ○ A nurse may not be responsible for the payment of damages unless the weight of the evidence shows that the care provided was not in accordance with the standards of practice.
        - ○ The failure to meet the standard of care must be a cause of the injury, and the injury must be permanent and/or have resulted in death.
- The chain of command should be written in institutional protocol.
    - • *Chain of command* reflects the organizational chart from the staff nurse to the chief nursing and medical officers.
    - • Some reasons for using the chain of command are:
        - ○ Provider does not respond to calls or pages.
        - ○ Provider shows signs of impairment.
        - ○ Provider's actions will potentially cause patient endangerment.
        - ○ Provider exhibits behavior that is unprofessional or threatening.

Nursing Interventions

- Use the chain of command.
- Follow all institutional policies, procedures, and standards of care.
- Objectively document all actions and interactions and the time they occur and include specific details of what is being reported to the provider.
  Example: At 12:20 p.m., the nurse notified Dr. Jones of FHR of 60 bpm × 90 seconds with no response to interventions. The nurse requested Dr. Jones to the bedside for immediate evaluation of the FHR tracing. At 12:25 p.m., the nurse paged Dr. Jones for FHR of 60 bpm × 390 seconds, with no response from Dr. Jones. The nurse then called Dr. Smith for immediate evaluation of FHR tracing.

POP QUIZ 6.3

A nurse is caring for a patient with a category III FHR tracing. The nurse calls the provider and leaves a message, but the provider does not respond. What is a priority for the nurse?

POP QUIZ 6.4

A nurse is caring for a patient with a category III FHR tracing. The nurse calls the provider. The provider does not respond to numerous attempts to call, but the nurse continues to call the provider and does not use the chain of command and call the next person in charge. What is the legal implication for the nurse?

PATIENT SAFETY

Overview

- Patient safety is an essential component of commitment to the provision of optimal healthcare.
- A *patient safety event* is any event or action that leads to, or has the potential to lead to, a worsened patient outcome related to the event or action. Events may be related to systems, operations, drug administration, or any clinical aspect of patient care.
- Communication is an essential component of patient safety.
  - Accurate, clear communication contributes to patient safety.
  - The healthcare team may use a variety of communication tools and techniques to facilitate accurate, clear, and concise communication.
  - Examples of effective communication tools and techniques include:
    - *Callout:* Conveys critical information to a larger group of people efficiently, directing the information to a specific individual.
    - *Closed-loop communication:* Ensures the recipient has understood the sender's information correctly.
    - *SBAR:* Used to request help in emergencies in which information needs to be conveyed quickly; briefly reports the *situation*, *background*, *assessment*, and *recommendation* from the provider
    - *CUS tool:* Important in communicating with the provider on what the specific issue is:
      - I am Concerned!
      - I am Uncomfortable!
      - This is a Safety issue!

(continued)

Overview *(continued)*

- Debriefing is an important part of all patient safety events.
- Debriefing is confidential and uses a nonjudgmental approach.
- Debriefing should be done immediately (or as soon as possible) after the safety event; all team members involved should debrief to discuss what went well and what could be improved as a team.
- Debriefing is also used to provide support to other team members.
- There is no finger pointing or singling out of team members during debriefing.
- Important steps to improve patient safety include:
  - Continuously review FHR tracings to maintain competence.
  - Implement recommended safe medication practices.
  - Improve communication among healthcare providers.
  - Improve communication with patients and family members.
  - Make safety a priority in every aspect of practice.
  - Practice for emergencies by performing simulations.
  - Recognize patients as full partners in care.
  - Reduce the likelihood of surgical errors by using a surgery checklist, ensuring a time out has been called, and ensuring that the surgical site has been marked.
  - Use teamwork and collaboration in the care of a patient.
- *Just culture* holds organizations accountable for the systems they have designed. In addition, just culture holds the organization accountable for responding to the behaviors of its employees in a manner that is both fair and just.
  - Adopt and develop safe practices that reduce the likelihood of system failures that can cause adverse outcomes. Most medication errors can be linked to a system failure—for example, care that is out of the nurse-to-patient ratio.
  - Ensure that instances of adverse outcomes or failure to follow safety protocols are investigated fairly and openly.
  - Ensure that nurses feel empowered to speak up when they are uncomfortable with an FHR tracing.
  - Identify and study the patterns and causes of error occurrence within delivery.
  - Identify FHR tracings that are not interpreted correctly. It is acceptable for the nurse to ask others to review an FHR tracing when uncertain of what is occurring.
- Just culture recognizes that some human error is inevitable.
- Just culture requires that nurses and providers recognize that the potential for errors exists.
- Just culture requires a learning environment that encourages disclosure and exchange of information in the event of errors, near misses, and adverse outcomes.
- Just culture recognizes the responsibility of all healthcare providers to follow safe practices and to avoid at-risk behaviors.
- Simulations are essential to enhance team skills in the OB setting.
  - Simulations should include all multidisciplinary team members.
  - Simulations should occur in a safe environment for learning and practice.
  - Simulations improve the safety of the patient, fetus, and newborn, as well as enhance teamwork and communication among the healthcare team.
  - Simulations promote interprofessional education and collaboration.

- Debriefing after simulation enhances team performance and improves clinician behavior and technical skills, as well as clinical performance and overall patient care. Simulations should offer opportunities for staff to ask questions and seek clarification as needed.

Nursing Interventions

- Communicate accurately and clearly using recognized tools and techniques.
- Debrief after each event.
- Report all patient safety events.
- Use the chain of command.

NURSING PEARL

Patient safety measures should be ongoing. All nurses and providers should use safe practices and encourage others to do so.

POP QUIZ 6.5

After a neonatal code in the operating room, team members discuss what went well and what could be improved. What is this an example of?

QUALITY IMPROVEMENT

Overview

- QI is a framework used to help improve healthcare and care of the patient.
- Concepts of QI include:
  - Establishing a culture of quality in your area
  - Determining and prioritizing potential areas for improvement
  - Collecting and analyzing data
  - Communicating results
  - Committing to ongoing evaluation
  - Spreading successes: Sharing lessons learned with others
- Determine what needs improvement by collecting and using benchmark data. Some examples include:
  - Breastfeeding rates
  - Catheter-associated urinary tract infection rates
  - Falls
  - Neonatal birth traumas
  - Nulliparous term singleton vertex cesarean section rates
- Ensure QI:
  - Implement evidence-based guidelines.
  - Improve outcomes.
  - Use standardization within QI to decrease deviation in results.
- Use these best practices when implementing QI projects:
  - Place a priority on encouraging communication, engagement, and participation for all of the stakeholders affected by the QI process.
  - Start with a small multidisciplinary team that is vested.
  - Start with small-scale changes.

(continued)

Overview *(continued)*

- Use a standardized process, such as the PDSA cycle, to implement QI projects or measures:
  - Plan: Determine what needs improving and how to make the improvement.
  - Do: Implement the change that is needed.
  - Study: Monitor the implementation and determine what changes are needed.
  - Act: Make appropriate changes as needed.

 ALERT!

It is important to note that hospital payments from insurance companies may be based on outcomes from quality data.

Nursing Interventions

- Follow evidence-based guidelines.
- Implement a QI project and monitor clinical activity through observation and collection of data.
- Use standardization when possible.
- Include stakeholders in the process.
- Report the effects of changes that were implemented.
- Track progress of the implementation process.

 POP QUIZ 6.6

What is the name of the process that can be used when implementing a QI project?

RESOURCES

Agency for Healthcare Research and Quality. (2020). *Section 4: Ways to approach the quality improvement process.* https://www.ahrq.gov/cahps/quality-improvement/improvement-guide/4-approach-qi-process/index.html

Agency for Healthcare Research and Quality. (2021a). *Approach to improving patient safety: Communication.* https://psnet.ahrq.gov/perspective/approach-improving-patient-safety-communication

Agency for Healthcare Research and Quality. (2021b). *CUS Tool - Improving communication and teamwork in the surgical environment module.* https://www.ahrq.gov/hai/tools/ambulatory-surgery/sections/implementation/training-tools/cus-tool.html

American Academy of Family Physicians. (n.d.). *Basics of quality improvement.* https://www.aafp.org/family-physician/practice-and-career/managing-your-practice/quality-improvement-basics.html

American College of Obstetricians and Gynecologists. (2007, Reaffirmed 2016). Ethical decision making in obstetrics and gynecology. *Obstetrics & Gynecology, 110*(6), 1479–1487. https://doi.org/10.1097/01.aog.0000291573.09193.36

American College of Obstetricians and Gynecologist. (2009). Patient safety in obstetrics and gynecology. *Obstetrics & Gynecology, 114*(6), 1424–1427. https://doi.org/10.1097/aog.0b013e3181c6f90e

Austin, N., Goldhaber-Fiebert, S., Daniels, K., Arafeh, J., Grenon, V., Welle, D., & Lipman, S. (2017). Building comprehensive strategies for obstetric safety: Simulation drills and communication. *Obstetric Anesthesia Digest, 37*(2), 61–62. https://doi.org/10.1097/01.aoa.0000515726.29190.ef

Birth Injury Help Center. (2021). *How long do you have to file a birth injury malpractice lawsuit?* https://www.birthinjuryhelpcenter.org/birth-injury-statute-of-limitations.html

Brigham and Women Faulkner Hospital.(2021). *What is just culture? Changing the way we think about errors to improve patient safety and staff satisfaction.* https://www.brighamandwomensfau lkner.org/about-bwfh/news/what-is-just-culture-changing-the-way-we-think-about-errors-to-improve-patient-safety-and-staff-satisfaction

Centers for Medicare & Medicaid Services. (2021). *Quality measurement and quality improvement.* U.S. Department of Health and Human Services, Centers for Medicare and Medicaid Services. https://www.cms.gov/Medicare/Quality-Initiatives-Patient-Assessment-Instruments/MMS/ Quality-Measure-and-Quality-Improvement

Cheng, A., Grant, V., Dieckmann, P., Arora, S., Robinson, T., & Eppich, W. (2015). Faculty development for simulation programs: Five issues for the future of debriefing training. *Simulation in Healthcare: The Journal of the Society for Simulation in Healthcare, 10*(4), 217–222. https://doi.or g/10.1097/SIH.0000000000000090. https://journals.lww.com/simulationinhealthcare/pages/article viewer.aspx?year=2015&issue=08000&article=00004&type=Fulltext

Harder, N. (2018). The value of simulation in health care: The obvious, the tangential, and the obscure. *Clinical Simulation in Nursing, 15,* 73–P74. https://doi.org/10.1016/j.ecns.2017.12.004. https://www.nursingsimulation.org/article/S1876-1399(17)30357-2/fulltext

Lippke, S., Derksen, C., Keller, F. M., Kötting, L., Schmiedhofer, M., & Welp, A. (2021). Effectiveness of communication interventions in obstetrics—A systematic review. *International Journal of Environmental Research and Public Health, 18*(5), 2616. https://doi.org/10.3390/ijerph18052616

OPLN Law. (2020). *Substandard quality of care: What you need to know.* https://lawnj.net/information /substandard-care/

7

TRACINGS ANALYSIS PRACTICE

PATIENT CASE STUDIES

Read the following case studies and use the FHR tracings to answer the questions.

Case Study 7.1

A 21-year-old patient is being evaluated for the first time. Based on the patient's subjective report, it is suspected that the patient is at 39 weeks' gestation. The FHR tracing is shown in Figure 7.1. Interpret the tracing and determine the priority interventions, if any, for the nurse caring for this patient.

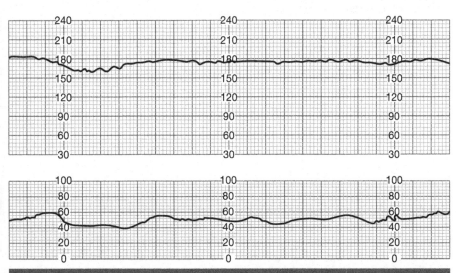

Figure 7.1

Source: Nye, R. (2019). *Essentials of fetal heart rate monitoring.* Springer Publishing Company.
doi:10.1891/9780826174246.0006

Heart rate:
FHR category:
Variability:
Acceleration (Y/N):
Deceleration (Y/N):
Type of deceleration:

Answers

Heart rate: 180

FHR category: II

Variability: Minimal

Acceleration (Y/N): N

Deceleration (Y/N): Y

Type of deceleration: Late

The tracing shows the presence of tachycardia, minimal variability, and late decelerations, indicating that the fetus is oxygen deprived. The priority nursing interventions include the following:

- Notify the provider.
- Place an IV.
- Start an IV fluid bolus infusion (normal saline or lactated Ringer's solution).
- Place patient on side.
- Administer oxygen.
- Prepare for emergent delivery.

Case Study 7.2

A 29-year-old patient is in labor. The patient's cervix measures 6 cm dilated. Butorphanol and promethazine were administered 30 minutes ago for pain relief. Interpret the FHR tracing shown in Figure 7.2 and determine the most appropriate nursing intervention, if any.

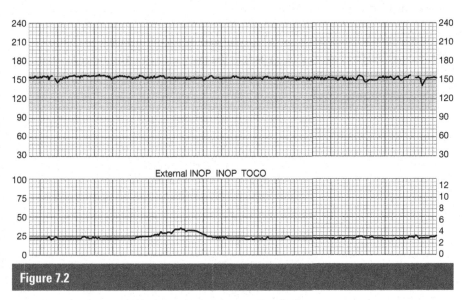

Figure 7.2

Source: Nye, R. (2019). *Essentials of fetal heart rate monitoring.* Springer Publishing Company. doi:10.1891/9780826174246.0006

Heart rate:
FHR category:
Variability:
Acceleration (Y/N):
Deceleration (Y/N):
Type of deceleration:

Answers
Heart rate: 150
FHR category: II
Variability: Minimal
Acceleration (Y/N): N
Deceleration (Y/N): N
Type of deceleration: None
No intervention is required. This is an expected finding after a patient has received butorphanol because narcotics can cause a decrease in the variability and frequency of accelerations.

Case Study 7.3

A 33-year-old patient at 40 weeks' and 2 days' gestation has been administered oxytocin for induction of labor. The FHR tracing is shown in Figure 7.3. Interpret the tracing and determine what, if any, nursing interventions are needed.

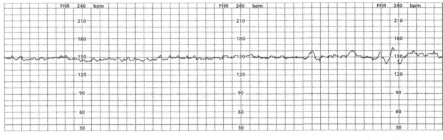

11:40

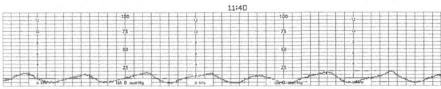

Figure 7.3

Source: Murray, M., Huelsmann, G., & Koperski, N. (2019). *Essentials of fetal and uterine monitoring.* Springer Publishing Company.

Heart rate:

FHR category:

Variability:

Acceleration (Y/N):

Deceleration (Y/N):

Type of deceleration:

Answers

Heart rate: 150

FHR category: II

Variability: Minimal

Acceleration (Y/N): N

Deceleration (Y/N): N

Type of deceleration: None

The tracing shows uterine tachysystole. The priority nursing interventions include the following:

- Discontinue the oxytocin.
- Reposition the patient.
- Administer an IV fluid bolus (normal saline or lactated Ringer's solution).

Case Study 7.4

A 24-year-old patient received an epidural 10 minutes ago. The FHR tracing is pictured in Figure 7.4. Interpret the tracing and describe the required nursing interventions, if any.

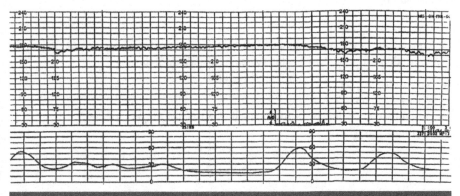

Figure 7.4

Source: Murray, M., Huelsmann, G., & Koperski, N. (2019). *Essentials of fetal and uterine monitoring.* Springer Publishing Company.

Heart rate:
FHR category:
Variability:
Acceleration (Y/N):
Deceleration (Y/N):
Type of deceleration:

Answers

Heart rate: 155

FHR category: II

Variability: Minimal

Acceleration (Y/N): N

Deceleration (Y/N): Y

Type of deceleration: Late

The tracing shows late decelerations, most likely caused by patient hypotension due to the epidural administration. Nursing interventions include the following:

- Notify the provider.
- Place patient on side.
- Administer an IV fluid bolus (normal saline or lactated Ringer's solution).
- Administer oxygen.

Case Study 7.5

A 22-year-old full-term patient is placed on the monitor. It is the patient's first pregnancy. The FHR tracing is shown in Figure 7.5. Interpret the tracing, determine the patient's FHR, and describe what the interpretation indicates is occurring. List any nursing interventions that are required.

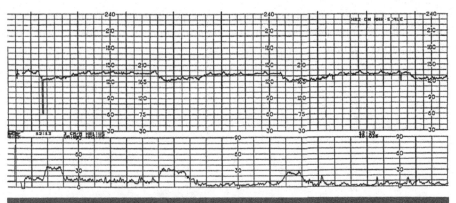

Figure 7.5

Source: Murray, M., Huelsmann, G., & Koperski, N. (2019). *Essentials of fetal and uterine monitoring.* Springer Publishing Company.

Heart rate:
FHR category:
Variability:
Acceleration (Y/N):
Deceleration (Y/N):
Type of deceleration:

Answers
Heart rate: 135
FHR category: I
Variability: Moderate
Acceleration (Y/N): N
Deceleration (Y/N): Y
Type of deceleration: Early
The tracing shows early decelerations, which are an expected finding indicating that labor is progressing. The nurse should continue to monitor the patient, but no other interventions are necessary at this time.

Case Study 7.6

A 19-year-old patient of unknown gestation is being evaluated for abdominal pain and to rule out contractions. The patient has no history of previous prenatal care and shows signs of substance use. Interpret the patient's FHR tracing in Figure 7.6, describe the likely cause, and indicate the priority nursing interventions, if any.

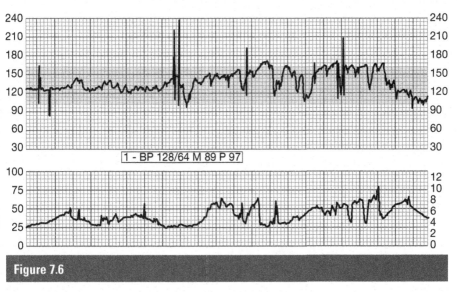

Figure 7.6

Source: Nye, R. (2019). *Essentials of fetal heart rate monitoring.* Springer Publishing Company. doi:10.1891/9780826174246.0006

Heart rate:
FHR category:
Variability:
Acceleration (Y/N):
Deceleration (Y/N):
Type of deceleration:

Answers
Heart rate: 125
FHR category: II
Variability: Marked
Acceleration (Y/N): Y
Deceleration (Y/N): N
Type of deceleration: None
The FHR tracing may indicate substance use. The priority nursing actions are to initiate monitoring of the patient and the fetus and to notify the provider.

Case Study 7.7

A 32-year-old patient who is 39 weeks' and 6 days' gestation presents in labor and requests an epidural. Interpret the patient's FHR tracing in Figure 7.7 and determine whether the fetus is acidotic. What nursing interventions, if any, are required?

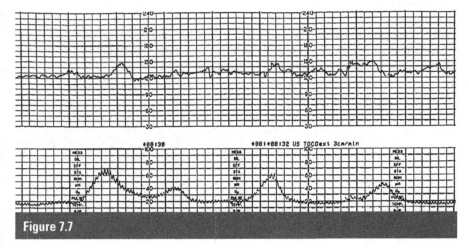

Figure 7.7

Source: Murray, M., Huelsmann, G., & Koperski, N. (2019). *Essentials of fetal and uterine monitoring.* Springer Publishing Company.

Heart rate:

FHR category:

Variability:

Acceleration (Y/N):

Deceleration (Y/N):

Type of deceleration:

Answers
Heart rate: 130
FHR category: I
Variability: Moderate
Acceleration (Y/N): Y
Deceleration (Y/N): N
Type of deceleration: None
This is a category I FHR tracing with a normal baseline, moderate variability, and accelerations present, indicating a nonacidotic fetus. No nursing interventions are currently required, but the nurse should continue to monitor per protocol.

Case Study 7.8

A patient received oxytocin to augment labor. Interpret the patient's FHR tracing in Figure 7.8 and indicate any required nursing interventions.

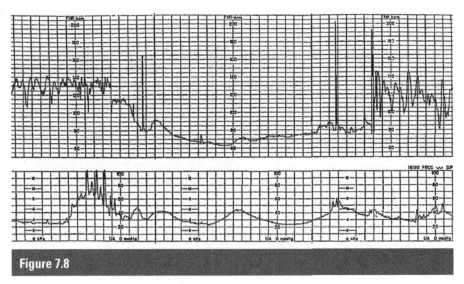

Figure 7.8

Source: Murray, M., Huelsmann, G., & Koperski, N. (2019). *Essentials of fetal and uterine monitoring.* Springer Publishing Company.

Heart rate:

FHR category:

Variability:

Acceleration (Y/N):

Deceleration (Y/N):

Type of deceleration:

Answers
Heart rate: Indeterminate
FHR category: II
Variability: Marked
Acceleration (Y/N): N
Deceleration (Y/N): Y
Type of deceleration: Prolonged
The FHR reveals a prolonged deceleration. The deceleration is classified as prolonged because it lasts longer than 2 minutes but less than 10 minutes. The prolonged deceleration is likely caused by uterine tachysystole. Nursing interventions include the following:

• Notify the provider.
• Discontinue the oxytocin.
• Administer an IV fluid bolus (normal saline or lactated Ringer's solution).
• Administer oxygen.
• Reposition the patient.

Case Study 7.9

A patient is being induced with oxytocin at 40 weeks' and 4 days' gestation. Interpret the patient's FHR tracing (Figure 7.9) and identify the area of greatest concern.

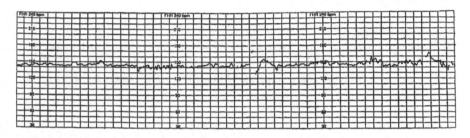

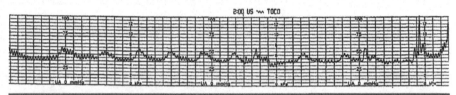

Figure 7.9

Source: Murray, M., Huelsmann, G., & Koperski, N. (2019). *Essentials of fetal and uterine monitoring.* Springer Publishing Company.

Heart rate:

FHR category:

Variability:

Acceleration (Y/N):

Deceleration (Y/N):

Type of deceleration:

Answers
Heart rate: 145
FHR category: I
Variability: Moderate
Acceleration (Y/N): Y
Deceleration (Y/N): N
Type of deceleration: None
The FHR tracing indicates uterine tachysystole, which leads to decreased fetal oxygenation and must be corrected. The nurse should discontinue the oxytocin, administer an IV fluid bolus (normal saline or lactated Ringer's solution), and notify the provider.

Case Study 7.10

A patient in labor receives an epidural. The FHR tracing in Figure 7.10 is obtained 10 minutes later. Interpret the tracing and identify any priority nursing interventions.

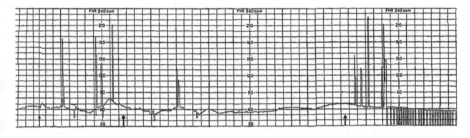

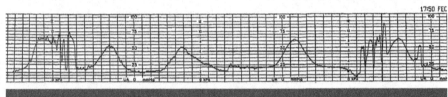

Figure 7.10

Source: Murray, M., Huelsmann, G., & Koperski, N. (2019). *Essentials of fetal and uterine monitoring.* Springer Publishing Company.

Heart rate:
FHR category:
Variability:
Acceleration (Y/N):
Deceleration (Y/N):
Type of deceleration:

Answers
Heart rate: 60 (bradycardia)
FHR category: III
Variability: Minimal
Acceleration (Y/N): Y
Deceleration (Y/N): N
Type of deceleration: None
This FHR tracing indicates fetal bradycardia, most likely due to maternal hypotension after epidural anesthesia. The nurse should do the following:

- Call the provider to the bedside immediately.
- Discontinue oxytocin.
- Administer oxygen.
- Administer an IV fluid bolus (normal saline or lactated Ringer's solution).
- Reposition the patient.

Case Study 7.11

A 17-year-old patient arrives via ambulance with severe abdominal pain and vaginal bleeding. The patient is at 32 weeks' gestation and has a history of substance use. What category is the FHR tracing (Figure 7.11), and what is the likely cause? What nursing interventions, if any, are necessary?

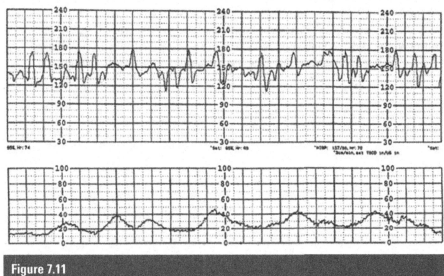

Figure 7.11

Source: Nye, R. (2019). *Essentials of fetal heart rate monitoring.* Springer Publishing Company. doi:10.1891/9780826174246.0006

Heart rate:
FHR category:
Variability:
Acceleration (Y/N):
Deceleration (Y/N):
Type of deceleration:

Answers
Heart rate: Indeterminate
FHR category: II
Variability: Marked
Acceleration (Y/N): N
Deceleration (Y/N): N
Type of deceleration: None
Because of the history of substance use; the painful, rigid abdomen; and the frequent contractions, the most likely cause is a placental abruption. Nursing interventions include placing the patient on their side, administering an IV fluid bolus (normal saline or lactated Ringer's solution), administering oxygen, notifying the provider, and preparing for emergent delivery.

Case Study 7.12

A 24-year-old patient at 41 weeks' gestation is being evaluated for reported decreased fetal movement since waking up this morning. Interpret the FHR tracing in Figure 7.12 and identify the priority nursing interventions, if any.

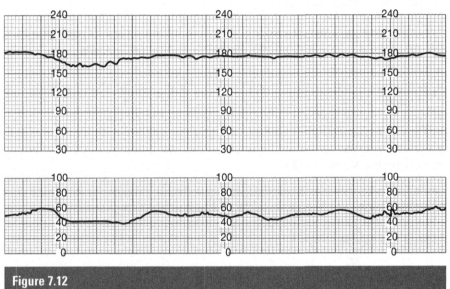

Figure 7.12

Source: Nye, R. (2019). *Essentials of fetal heart rate monitoring.* Springer Publishing Company. doi:10.1891/9780826174246.0006

Heart rate:
FHR category:
Variability:
Acceleration (Y/N):
Deceleration (Y/N):
Type of deceleration:

Answers

Heart rate: 180

FHR category: II

Variability: Minimal

Acceleration (Y/N): N

Deceleration (Y/N): Y

Type of deceleration: Late

The FHR tracing confirms decreased fetal movement, which indicates that the fetus is being deprived of oxygen. The nurse's priority interventions include the following:

- Notify the provider.
- Activate the emergency call system for other healthcare team members to provide immediate assistance.
- Administer an IV fluid bolus (normal saline or lactated Ringer's solution).
- Place patient on side.
- Administer oxygen.
- Prepare for emergent delivery.

Case Study 7.13

A patient presents for induction of labor at 41 weeks' and 2 days' gestation. It is the patient's first pregnancy. The cervical examination is 2 cm/30%/-3. The provider orders a cervical ripening agent. Interpret the FHR tracing in Figure 7.13 and indicate the next step for the nurse.

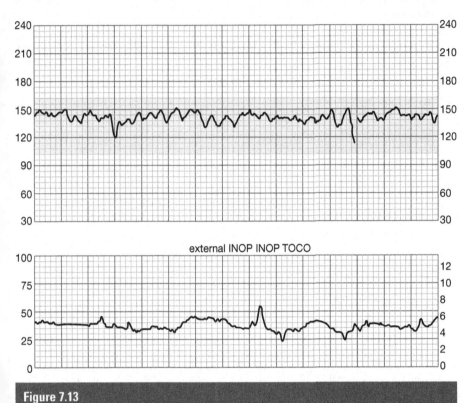

Figure 7.13

Source: Nye, R. (2019). *Essentials of fetal heart rate monitoring.* Springer Publishing Company. doi:10.1891/9780826174246.0006

Heart rate:

FHR category:

Variability:

Acceleration (Y/N):

Deceleration (Y/N):

Type of deceleration:

Answers

Heart rate: 140

FHR category: I

Variability: Moderate

Acceleration (Y/N): N

Deceleration (Y/N): N

Type of deceleration: None

The FHR is category I. The next step for the nurse is to administer the cervical ripening agent as ordered.

Case Study 7.14

A patient has had ruptured membranes for 32 hours. The patient was induced with oxytocin and is now dilated to 10 cm and is pushing. Interpret the patient's FHR tracing (Figure 7.14), and indicate the likely cause of the findings. What nursing interventions, if any, are required?

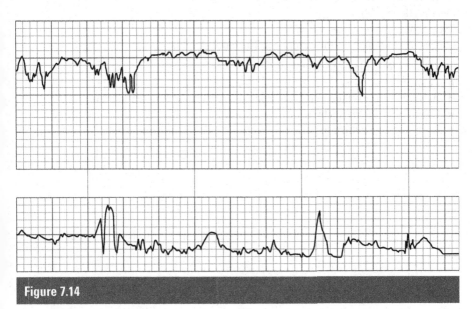

Figure 7.14

Source: National Certification Corporation. (2021). *Fetal assessment and safe labor management.* Appendix A. https://www.nccwebsite.org/content/documents/cms/2016_ncc_monograph_free_version.pdf. (NCC does not sponsor or endorse this resource, nor does it have a proprietary relationship with Springer Publishing Company.)

Heart rate:
FHR category:
Variability:
Acceleration (Y/N):
Deceleration (Y/N):
Type of deceleration:

Answers
Heart rate: 180
FHR category: II
Variability: Moderate
Acceleration (Y/N): N
Deceleration (Y/N): Y
Type of deceleration: Late, variable
The patient may have chorioamnionitis. The nurse should:

- Monitor the patient's temperature.
- Reposition the patient.
- Administer an IV fluid bolus (normal saline or lactated Ringer's solution).
- Discontinue the oxytocin.
- Encourage the patient to push with every second or third contraction.

Case Study 7.15

A 30-year-old patient with preeclampsia is admitted for evaluation of new-onset headache and reported decreased fetal movement. Interpret the initial FHR tracing in Figure 7.15, and identify the priority nursing interventions, if any.

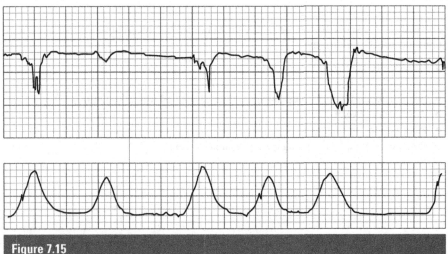

Figure 7.15

Source: National Certification Corporation. (2021). *Fetal assessment and safe labor management.* Appendix C. https:// www.nccwebsite.org/content/documents/cms/2016_ncc_monograph_free_version.pdf. (NCC does not sponsor or endorse this resource, nor does it have a proprietary relationship with Springer Publishing Company.)

Heart rate:
FHR category:
Variability:
Acceleration (Y/N):
Deceleration (Y/N):
Type of deceleration:

Answers

Heart rate: 150

FHR category: III

Variability: Absent

Acceleration (Y/N): N

Deceleration (Y/N): Y

Type of deceleration: Variable

The FHR is a category III tracing that requires immediate intervention. Nursing interventions include the following:

- Call the provider.
- Start an IV.
- Administer an IV fluid bolus (normal saline or lactated Ringer's solution).
- Administer oxygen.
- Place patient on side.
- Prepare the patient for an emergency cesarean section.

Case Study 7.16

A patient is admitted for cervical ripening before induction. The provider sees the FHR and provides fetal scalp stimulation with a vaginal examination. What are some possible causes for the FHR shown in Figure 7.16, and what interventions are needed, if any?

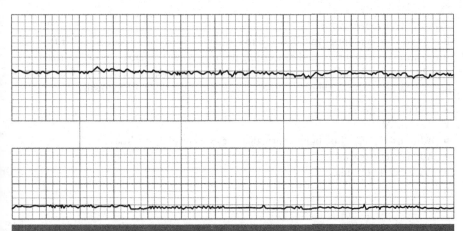

Figure 7.16

Source: National Certification Corporation. (2021). *Fetal assessment and safe labor management.* Appendix C. https://www.nccwebsite.org/content/documents/cms/2016_ncc_monograph_free_version.pdf. (NCC does not sponsor or endorse this resource, nor does it have a proprietary relationship with Springer Publishing Company.)

Heart rate:
FHR category:
Variability:
Acceleration (Y/N):
Deceleration (Y/N):
Type of deceleration:

Answers

Heart rate: 140
FHR category: II
Variability: Minimal
Acceleration (Y/N): N
Deceleration (Y/N): N
Type of deceleration: None

It is important to monitor the FHR and the patient because no acceleration after fetal scalp stimulation is an abnormal and concerning finding. While the fetus may be in a sleep cycle, possible concerning causes of no acceleration after fetal scalp stimulation include a neurologic or cardiac issue or hypoxia. Nursing interventions include the following:

- Call the provider.
- Start an IV.
- Administer an IV fluid bolus (normal saline or lactated Ringer's solution).
- Administer oxygen.
- Place patient on side.

Case Study 7.17

A 28-year-old patient with Sjogren's syndrome is admitted in labor at 39 weeks. Interpret the FHR in Figure 7.17, identify the likely cause of the tracing, and list any necessary nursing interventions.

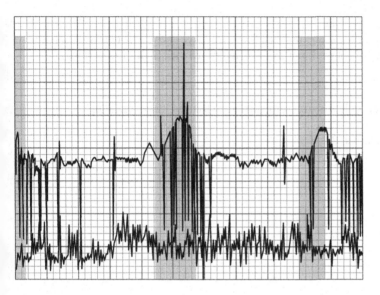

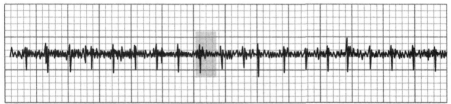

Figure 7.17

Source: Lakhno, I., Behar, J. A., Oster, J., Shulgin, V., Ostras, O., & Andreotti, F. (2017). The use of non-invasive fetal electrocardiography in diagnosing second-degree fetal atrioventricular block. *Maternal Health, Neonatology and Perinatology.* Figure 3. https://mhnpjournal.biomedcentral.com/articles/10.1186/s40748-017-0053-1. DOI 10.1186/s40748-017-0053-1. https://creativecommons.org/licenses/by/4.0/

Heart rate:
FHR category:
Variability:
Acceleration (Y/N):
Deceleration (Y/N):
Type of deceleration:

Answers

Heart rate: 120

FHR category: I

Variability: Moderate

Acceleration (Y/N): Y

Deceleration (Y/N): N

Type of deceleration: None

The FHR is reactive but shows dropped beats. The most likely cause of this tracing is heart block owing to Sjogren's syndrome. Nursing interventions include the following:

- Call the provider.
- Start an IV.
- Administer an IV fluid bolus (normal saline or lactated Ringer's solution).
- Administer oxygen.
- Place patient on side.

Case Study 7.18

A 20-year-old patient is 10 cm dilated and begins pushing. Interpret the patient's FHR tracing (Figure 7.18), and identify the most appropriate nursing interventions.

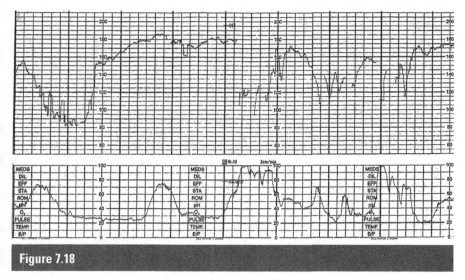

Figure 7.18

Source: Murray, M., Huelsmann, G., & Koperski, N. (2019). *Essentials of fetal and uterine monitoring.* Springer Publishing Company.

Heart rate:

FHR category:

Variability:

Acceleration (Y/N):

Deceleration (Y/N):

Type of deceleration:

Answers

Heart rate: Indeterminate

FHR category: II

Variability: Indeterminate

Acceleration (Y/N): N

Deceleration (Y/N): Y

Type of deceleration: Variable

Nursing interventions include the following:

- Reposition the patient.
- Administer an IV fluid bolus (normal saline or lactated Ringer's solution).
- Administer oxygen.
- Encourage pushing every second or third contraction to allow for fetal oxygenation.
- If the FHR remains the same, the provider should be notified.

Case Study 7.19

A 29-year-old patient at 40+1 weeks' gestation has been in labor for 28 hours and has not received any opioids. The FHR has been category II for more than 10 hours. The FHR tracing is shown in Figure 7.19. What nursing interventions, if any, are needed?

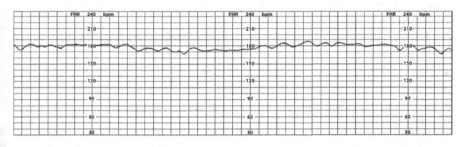

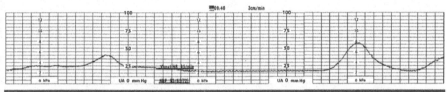

Figure 7.19

Source: Murray, M., Huelsmann, G., & Koperski, N.(2019). *Essentials of fetal and uterine monitoring.* Springer Publishing Company.

Heart rate:
FHR category:
Variability:
Acceleration (Y/N):
Deceleration (Y/N):
Type of deceleration:

Answers

Heart rate: 180
FHR category: II
Variability: N/A
Acceleration (Y/N): N
Deceleration (Y/N): N
Type of deceleration: None

The FHR reveals a sinusoidal pattern and requires immediate attention. The nurse should do the following:

- Call the provider.
- Start an IV.
- Administer an IV fluid bolus (normal saline or lactated Ringer's solution).
- Administer oxygen.

Case Study 7.20

The nurse performs all of the interventions described in Case Study 7.19. The tracing remains the same. What can the nurse expect to occur next?

Answer

The nurse can expect the provider to perform a cesarean section if vaginal delivery is not immediately pending.

RESOURCES

Garite, T. J., & Simpson, K. R. (2011). Intrauterine resuscitation during labor. *Clinical Obstetrics & Gynecology, 54*(1), 28–39. https://doi.org/10.1097/grf.0b013e31820a062b

Lakhno, I., Behar, J. A., Oster, J., Shulgin, V., Ostras, O., & Andreotti, F. (2017). *The use of non-invasive fetal electrocardiography in diagnosing second-degree fetal atrioventricular block. Maternal Health, Neonatology and Perinatology, 14.* https://mhnpjournal.biomedcentral.com/articles/10.1186/s40748-017-0053-1

Murray, M., Huelsmann, G., & Koperski, N. (2019). *Essentials of fetal and uterine monitoring.* Springer Publishing Company.

National Certification Corporation. (2021). *Fetal assessment and safe labor management.* https://www.nccwebsite.org/content/documents/cms/2016_ncc_monograph_free_version.pdf

Nye, R. (2019). *Essentials of fetal heart rate monitoring.* Springer Publishing. https://doi.org/10.1891/9780826174246.0006

8

POP QUIZ ANSWERS

CHAPTER 2

POP QUIZ 2.1

The best way to improve uteroplacental circulation is to stabilize maternal–fetal oxygen status. To stabilize maternal–fetal oxygen status, the nurse should change the position of the patient, administer an IV fluid bolus, and administer supplemental oxygen as needed.

CHAPTER 3

POP QUIZ 3.1

The nurse should call the provider to the bedside.

POP QUIZ 3.2

The amniotic sac must be broken, which means there is an increased risk of infection.

POP QUIZ 3.3

Uterine tachysystole is defined as more than five contractions in 10 minutes.

POP QUIZ 3.4

The fetus may be in a sleep cycle. Vibroacoustic stimulation can be performed to attempt to wake the fetus out of the sleep cycle.

POP QUIZ 3.5

It is not normal. It is normal for *decelerations* to occur with pushing. The nurse should continue to monitor the fetus and also monitor the patient's pulse. If there still appear to be fetal accelerations, an FSE may be requested.

CHAPTER 4

POP QUIZ 4.1

The nurse should change the patient's position, administer an IV fluid bolus, administer oxygen 8 to 10 L per nonrebreather mask, and call the provider. *Note:* Per institutional guidelines, the IV fluid bolus will be lactated Ringer's or normal saline.

POP QUIZ 4.2

Variability is the most important characteristic of fetal heart tracings in determining fetal well-being.

POP QUIZ 4.3

Variable decelerations may be resolved with amnioinfusion due to the decrease of cord compression.

CHAPTER 5

POP QUIZ 5.1

The concern for this patient would be at the maternal circulation step of the maternal–fetal oxygenation pathway. An interruption here can cause decreased cardiac output, altering fetal oxygenation.

POP QUIZ 5.2

Eclampsia is a possible diagnosis.

POP QUIZ 5.3

The nurse is attempting to prevent pulmonary edema.

POP QUIZ 5.4

The nurse could mention signs of preeclampsia (such as headache, blurred vision, epigastric pain, and swelling), eclampsia (seizures), or HELLP syndrome (abdominal pain).

POP QUIZ 5.5

The risk is for compression of the IVC, which can cause hypotension, late decelerations in the fetus, and possibly fetal death.

POP QUIZ 5.6

First, the nurse should call for help. Then, the nurse should insert a straight or Foley catheter into the bladder. It is likely that the bladder is filling or full and is displacing the uterus, causing the excessive bleeding.

POP QUIZ 5.7

The patient is likely experiencing an abruptio placentae. The nurse should call for help and a provider. The nurse should then prepare for an emergent cesarean section with full neonatal resuscitation. A urine drug screen (suspected cocaine) and a blood transfusion may be ordered.

POP QUIZ 5.8

The nurse should prepare for a possible shoulder dystocia by having extra nurses at the delivery, including one to care for the neonate. A stool should be available on each side of the bed in case suprapubic pressure is needed. A nurse should be assigned to document what happens at delivery.

CHAPTER 6

POP QUIZ 6.1

Respect for patient autonomy applies in this case. The nurse may feel that they do not have time to follow this evidence-based practice, but the patient has a right to it as long as the neonate is stable.

POP QUIZ 6.2

The principle of justice applies because the nurse is helping to ensure that underserved patients also receive adequate care.

POP QUIZ 6.3

The nurse must use the chain of command as determined by institutional policy. This means a call should be made to the next person in charge, and the nurse may need to go beyond that person if there is no response.

POP QUIZ 6.4

The nurse did not follow standard of care and could face legal action.

POP QUIZ 6.5

This is an example of debriefing.

POP QUIZ 6.6

The process is called PDSA (plan, do, study, act).

APPENDIX: ABBREVIATIONS

ABO	ABO blood group system
ACOG	American College of Obstetricians and Gynecologiststem
AORN	Association of periOperative Registered Nurses
AV	atrioventricular
AWHONN	Association of Women's Health, Obstetric and Neonatal Nurses
BMI	body mass index
BP	blood pressure
bpm	beats per minute
BPP	biophysical profile
CBC	complete blood count
COPD	chronic obstructive pulmonary disease
CST	contraction stress test
CUS	concerned, uncomfortable, safety
EFM	electronic fetal monitoring
EKG	electrocardiogram
FFP	fresh frozen plasma
FHR	fetal heart rate
FSE	fetal scalp electrode
GDM	gestational diabetes mellitus
HELLP	hemolysis, elevated liver enzymes, low platelet count
I/O	intake and output
IUGR	intrauterine growth restriction
IUPC	intrauterine pressure catheter
IV	intravenous
IVC	inferior vena cava
IVP	intravenous push
L&D	labor and delivery
NCC	National Certification Corporation
NSAID	nonsteroidal anti-inflammatory drug
OB	obstetric
PDSA	plan, do, study, act
PO	per os/by mouth
PPH	postpartum hemorrhage
QBL	quantitative blood loss
QI	quality improvement
RBC	red blood cell
SBAR	situation, background, assessment, recommendation
UA	umbilical artery
UV	umbilical vein

INDEX

abdominal trauma, 60
abruptio placenta, 60–61
  complete, 60
  partial, 60
acid–base result, 20
albuterol, 31
amnioinfusion, 12, 40, 58, 64, 128
amniotic fluid, 18, 19, 74
  volume, 18
amniotic sac, 23, 69, 127
amniotomy, 15
amplitude range, 28–31
anemia, 27, 45, 48, 53
anesthesia, 49, 50, 106
  epidural, 49
  spinal, 49
anesthetics, 29
anticonvulsant, 51, 57
antidote, 51
Apgar score, 21
arrest of labor, 73
arrhythmia, 42
  bradycardia, 42
    prolonged, 27
  pseudo-sinusoidal, 44–45
  sinusoidal, 44
  tachycardia, 43–44
    persistent, 27
asphyxia, 42
assessment
  biophysical profile, 18
    interpretation, 18
  biophysical profile: modified, 18–19
    interpretation, 19
  contraction stress test, 19
    interpretation, 19
  fetal movement, 20
    interpretation, 20
  fetal scalp stimulation, 23
    interpretation, 23

nonstress test, 16–18
  indications, 16
  nonreactive, 17
  reactive, 17
umbilical cord blood gas testing,
  20–21
  indications, 20–21
  interpretation, 21
  normal values, 21
uterine activity, 13–15
vibroacoustic stimulation, 22–23
auscultate, 48
auscultation, 15–16
autocorrelation algorithms, 12

barbiturates, 29
beta adrenergic receptor agonist, 57, 75
beta-blocker, 51
blood-brain barrier, 5
blood loss, 21, 49, 54, 70, 71
blood pressure, 39, 50–52, 57
BP. See blood pressure
BPP. See assessment, biophysical profile
breech, 35, 65

calcium channel blocker, 52, 57, 75
calcium gluconate, 51, 52
CBC. See complete blood count
C-EFM. See Electronic Fetal Monitoring
  Certification
cerebral palsy, 69
cervical ripening agent, 59, 111, 112
cesarean section, 30, 40, 43, 45, 49, 58, 62, 65, 66,
  72, 73, 78, 126, 129
chorioamnionitis, 14, 27, 43, 69, 114
circulation, 20, 47, 59, 127
  fetal, 5, 6
cocaine, 15, 32, 60, 129
complete blood count, 53, 54, 61
congenital anomalies, 27, 29

contraction, 9–16, 19, 34–36, 49, 55–57, 59, 73, 79, 108, 114, 122
  nadir, 36
corticosteroid, 57, 74, 75
critical nursing skills, 79
CST. *See* assessment, contraction stress test

dehydration, 49
  maternal, 59
diabetes, 38, 57, 60, 67, 68, 71–72
dilation, 13
  cervical, 65
ductus arteriosus, 5, 6
ductus venosus, 5, 6

effacement, 13
  cervical, 13
EFM. *See* electronic fetal monitoring
EKG. *See* electrocardiogram
electrocardiogram, 49, 119
electronic fetal monitoring, 9, 10
  tracing, 9
electronic fetal monitoring certification
  application, 2
electronic fetal monitoring certification
  recertification, 2
  requirements, 1
ethics, 7–8
  committee, 78
  ethical decision-making, 77
  principles, 77
    beneficence, 77
    justice, 77
    nonmaleficence, 77
    respect for patient autonomy, 77–78

fetal complications, 2, 27, 47, 80
  categories, 47
  environmental, 47–48
  fetus, 65–68
    acidosis, 65–67
    hypoxia, 65–67
    shoulder dystocia, 67–68
  labor, 73–75
    failure to progress, 73
    preterm, 74–75
  maternal blood flow, 48–56
    blood disorder, 48–49
    cardiac disease, 48–49
    chronic hypertension, 50
    eclampsia, 50
    gestational hypertension, 50
    HELLP syndrome, 50
    hemorrhage, 53–55
    hypotension, 49

    hypovolemia, 53–55
    inferior vena cava compression, 55–56
    preeclampsia, 50
  maternal respiratory system, 48
    respiratory depression, 48
  maternal seizure, 56–57
    focal, 56
    generalized, 56
  other maternal complications
    chorioamnionitis, 69
    diabetes mellitus, 71–72
    failure to progress, 73
    obesity, 72
  placenta, 60–62
    abruptio placenta, 60–61
    placental implantation, 61–62
  umbilical cord, 62–65
    compression, 63–64
    nuchal cord, 62–63
    prolapse, 64–65
  uterus, 58–60
    excessive uterine activity, 59–60
    uterine rupture, 58–59
fetal death, 10, 55, 129
fetal defect, 10
fetal distress, 10, 23, 29, 58
fetal heart block, 42
fetal heart rate, 2, 25–42
  acceleration, 32–33
    prolonged, 33
  baseline, 27–28
    abnormal, 27
  deceleration, 34–45
    early, 34–39
    episodic, 40
    late, 36–39
    periodic, 40
    prolonged, 41–42
    variable, 40
  tracing, 25–26
    category I, 25–26
    category II, 26
    category III, 26
  variability, 28–32
    absent, 29–30
    marked, 31–32
    minimal, 29–30
    moderate, 30–31
fetal kick count. *See* assessment, fetal movement
fetal monitoring
  artifact, 12–13
  continuous, 10
    high-risk patients, 10
  equipment failure, 13
    causes, 13

external monitor, 10–11
  Doppler ultrasound transducer, 10
  fetoscope, 10
  tocodynamometer, 11
intermittent, 10
internal monitor, 11–12
  fetal scalp electrode, 11
  intrauterine pressure catheter, 11
  membrane rupturing, 11
routine, 10
fetal scalp electrode, 11
FHR. *See* fetal heart rate
foramen ovale, 5
forceps, 71, 73
FSE. *See* fetal monitoring, internal monitor fetal
    scalp electrode

GDM. *See* gestational diabetes mellitus
gestation, 12, 16, 17, 32, 50, 74, 78, 87, 91, 97, 99,
    107, 111, 123
gestational diabetes mellitus, 71, 72
  A1, 71
  A2, 71

hematoma, 71
hemorrhage, 53–55
  postpartum, 70–71
hypertension, 36, 50–52, 56
hypoxemia, 29, 36, 37
hypoxic-ischemic encephalopathy, 10
hysterectomy, 62, 70

infection, 23, 69, 70, 73, 74, 83
  risk, 127
informed consent, 77
intrapartum fever, 21
intravenous fluid bolus, 5, 15, 30, 38, 47, 48, 53, 55,
    61, 62, 66, 71, 92, 102, 104, 106, 108, 110,
    114, 116, 118, 120, 122, 124, 127, 128
intravenous push, 51, 52
IUPC. *See* fetal monitoring, internal monitor,
    intrauterine pressure catheter
IVP. *See* intravenous push

labor, 10, 12, 14, 19, 34, 49, 55, 73–75
  dysfunctional, 14, 15
  induction, 14
  preterm, 57, 74–75
lactated Ringer's, 15, 42, 88, 92, 94, 104, 106, 108,
    110, 114, 116, 118, 120, 124, 128
legal implication, 77, 81
legal issues, 77
  chain of command, 80
  lawsuits, 79, 80
  negligence, 80
    breach of duty, 80

causation, 80
  damages, 80
  duty, 80
  standard of care, 79–80
    substandard intrapartal care, 79

maneuver, 11, 68
  desperation, 68
  Gaskin, 68
  Leopold's, 11, 67
  posterior axilla sling traction, 68
  Rubin, 68
  Woods screw, 68
  Zavanelli, 68
maternal cardiac, 10, 48–49, 53
maternal position
  hands and knees, 63
  lateral, 47, 53, 63
  lateral recumbent, 16
  left lateral, 49, 53, 55
  right lateral, 63
  semi-Fowler's, 16
  supine, 49, 55, 68
  Trendelenburg, 40, 65
metabolic acidosis, 10, 21, 23, 42, 43
methamphetamine, 32
multiple gestation, 12, 14, 16, 70, 74

narcotic, 29, 45, 90
National Certification Corporation, 1–3
nicotine, 32
nipple stimulation, 19
nonrebreather mask, 26, 27, 128
normal saline, 42, 88, 94, 102, 104, 106, 108, 110,
    114, 116, 118
NSAID, 57, 75
nuchal cord, 40, 62–63

oligohydramnios, 16, 17, 63
operative delivery. *See* cesarean section
operative vaginal delivery, 73, 74
oxygenation, 2, 5–7, 42, 47–49, 55, 56, 60, 64, 67,
    104, 128
  fetal, 2, 5–7, 19, 27, 47–49, 55, 60, 64, 104,
    128
    environmental conditions, 47
    phases, 5
  maternal, 5–7
  maternal blood flow, 7
  maternal respiratory system, 7
  maternal vasculature, 7
  placenta, 7
  umbilical cord, 7
  uterus, 7
oxytocin, 15, 19, 26, 30, 40, 42, 48, 49, 54, 55, 59, 70,
    73, 91, 92, 104, 106, 113, 114

phase of labor, 73
  active, 73
  prolonged latent, 73
phenothiazine, 29, 44
placenta abruptio, 21, 60–61
placenta accreta, 61
placenta incretaplacenta increta, 62
placental abruption. *See* placenta abruptio
placental infarction, 66
placental perfusion, 27, 53
placenta previa, 53
PPH. *See* hemorrhage, postpartum
preeclampsia, 10, 50–52, 56, 60, 66, 72, 128
pregestational diabetes mellitus, 71
  type 1, 72
  type 2, 72
premature fetus, 27, 29, 40
prostaglandin, 15, 49, 54, 55, 57
pulse oximetry, 12, 48
pushing, 12, 13, 40, 49, 59, 73, 113, 121, 127
  modification of, 47, 56, 64

QI. *See* quality improvement
quality improvement, 83–84
  best practices, 83
    PDSA cycle, 84
  concepts, 83
quantitative blood loss measurement, 53, 71

rapid fetal descent, 42
resting tone, 11, 14, 15, 59

safety
  communication
    callout, 81
    closed-loop, 81
    CUS tool, 81
    SBAR, 81

debriefing, 82
  patient safety event, 81, 82
  simulation, 82
seizure, 41, 47, 56–58, 128
semisynthetic ergot alkaloid
    derivative, 54
sleep cycle, 17, 29, 30, 118, 127
spontaneous labor, 15

terbutaline, 15, 31, 44
tranquilizer, 29
turtle sign, 67

UA. *See* umbilical artery
ultrasonographer, 18
umbilical cord compression, 39–41, 63–64
umbilical cord prolapse, 40, 41, 64–65
umbilical vein, 5, 21, 39
uterine activity, 2, 9, 13–15, 73
  excessive, 59–60
uterine artery embolization, 70
uterine compression suture, 70
uterine contraction, 9, 11–13, 19, 28, 33, 40, 53, 58, 73, 79
  abnormal, 2
    functional dystocia, 14
    tachysystole, 14
  duration, 14
  frequency, 14
  normal, 14
  strength, 14
uterine hyperactivity, 41
uterine rupture, 21, 41, 58–59, 67
uteroplacental insufficiency, 36
UV. *See* umbilical vein

vacuum, 71, 73
vasodilator, 52

Printed in the United States
by Baker & Taylor Publisher Services